Medical
Prediction Models

Chapman & Hall/CRC Biostatistics Series

Recently Published Titles

Medical Risk Prediction Models

With Ties to Machine Learning

Thomas A. Gerds
Michael W. Kattan

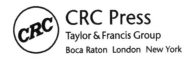

CRC Press
Taylor & Francis Group
Boca Raton London New York

CRC Press is an imprint of the
Taylor & Francis Group, an **informa** business

A CHAPMAN & HALL BOOK

First edition published 2021
by CRC Press
6000 Broken Sound Parkway NW, Suite 300, Boca Raton, FL 33487-2742

and by CRC Press
2 Park Square, Milton Park, Abingdon, Oxon, OX14 4RN

© 2021 Taylor & Francis Group, LLC

CRC Press is an imprint of Taylor & Francis Group, LLC

ISBN: 978-1-138-38447-7 (hbk)
ISBN: 978-1-138-38448-4 (ebk)

*To Mimi
and the gang.*

Contents

Foreword

Thomas Gerds and Michael Kattan are two researchers who live on the front lines of clinical prediction research and have extensive experience in the field. Their immersion into clinical research and close collaboration with clinician scientists gives them familiarity with clinical decision making, and they know how to communicate with clinicians. The methods presented in their book have wide applicability to clinical medicine. The emphasis on collaborating closely with physicians to formulate models is a proven approach to making models more relevant and reliable.

In an age where machine learning is being utilized with increasing frequency, the authors provide a nice overview of machine learning methods, fully recognizing advantages and disadvantages of this approach. Currently, many machine learning clinical prediction applications are being touted as providing more discriminating predictions than statistical models, but a good deal of this improvement in predictive discrimination comes at the cost of worse performance in terms of calibration accuracy (absolute predictive accuracy). Gerds and Kattan's emphasis on checking model calibration comes at a great time.

Many books and articles on clinical prediction give too much emphasis to all-or-nothing classification of patients into disease or outcome categories without grasping the importance of probabilistic reasoning in medicine. Many sources, especially ones involving machine learning, often use accuracy measures such as proportion of patients classified correctly, which when maximized actually leads to suboptimal decisions. Gerds and Kattan took a strongly supported position to emphasize probability accuracy scores such as the Brier score (mean squared error of prediction). Such scores are sensitive, place proper rewards on good predictions, and are not arbitrary. This was an excellent decision.

The attention to competing risks, because in most studies there are more than one possible clinical outcome, is a welcome addition to the clinical prediction literature.

One of the ways I evaluate a book is to check that out-of-date statistical methods or methods that do not represent best statistical practice are omitted. One of the things I most like about the book is the list of methods the authors purposefully excluded. These include risk thresholding, goodness-of-fit tests that arbitrarily categorize predicted risks, stepwise variable selection, reclassification tables using arbitrary risk thresholds, and graphical presentations that condition on the wrong variable (the outcome). The book not only covers a wide spectrum of very important topics but it also omits the right topics.

Frank E Harrell Jr.
September 2020

Preface

Everyone would like to build a medical risk prediction model and then "validate" it. There are many ways to make a model, and every modeling expert has preferences regarding the general approach and tuning. Our book is about the evaluation and comparison of medical risk prediction models, whether developed with machine learning, traditional statistical techniques, or other methods. What sets this book apart is the recognition that the evaluation of a medical risk prediction model, in isolation, is very difficult to do. Interpretation of prediction performance should always involve a benchmark, ideally that set by a rival prediction model. We should always be trying to predict more accurately today than we did yesterday and challenge the currently used models and guidelines. The cover art illustrates the medical future: patients consult the Internet and receive a predicted risk, such as 17%. The value 17% has a direct interpretation for the patient: if we had 100 patients exactly like you, we would expect 17 to have the outcome event within a given time span.

The only useful function of a statistician is to make predictions, and thus to provide a basis for action. – WE Deming

If you provide the same dataset to 10 different statisticians/modelers, you will receive 10 different prediction models, each yielding (to some degree) different predictions. Which one is best? The aim of this book is to empower you to be the fully informed referee of this competition. Our book is the platform upon which you should guide your judgment.

You will see that this book is designed to keep you out of trouble. The first big trap that many fall into is not recognizing the setting that they are in: binary outcome, time-until-event outcome, or competing risks. We provide clear lanes so that you choose the right one and stay in there, applying the methods appropriate for that lane. In short, time matters, and there are no events following death.

Our book provides a hands-on toolbox for medical risk prediction modeling. A central message is that simple estimates of odds ratios and hazard ratios with their corresponding null hypothesis tests should be replaced by data splitting and suitable performance metrics. Another key message is the proper treatment of time and competing risks when the prediction problem is defined. We emphasize that, in addition to the average performance of a model, individualized risk predictions need to be investigated and visualized.

But perhaps the most serious source of error lies in letting statistical procedures make decisions for you. – PI Good & JW Hardin

This helps to not overlook that a fancy modeling algorithm may produce a biologically implausible model with high average performance scores. Another highlight is the dependence of all this on the random seed. It seems that some researchers argue that the reason for setting the random seed is to achieve reproducibility of the results. However, the consequences of a medical risk prediction that depends on a specific random seed are terrible: the decision aid for a patient in a difficult situation of life should not depend on the favorite number (e.g., the random seed) of the data analyst.

Our book will help you put into practice what you might have read elsewhere, such as in the Transparent Reporting of a multivariable prediction model for Individual Prognosis or Diagnosis (TRIPOD) statement. We define "risk" precisely and contrast it with other terms such as hazard rates. Throughout the journey, we promote a collaboration between subject matter expert and biostatistician to fully realize the possibilities of effective statistical prediction models. Such a collaboration is behind the spirit of this book.

Mike learned about machine learning, prediction, and the many related issues from Louis Glorfeld. His way into the field was influenced by colleagues and mentors including J Robert Beck, Peter T Scardino, Ken Hess, Frank Harrell Jr., Glenn Heller, and Mithat Gonen. Thomas learned about medical risk prediction from Martin Schumacher and Erika Graf. Mike and Thomas were introduced to each other on a nice summer day in Prague. Our mutual friend, Donna Ankerst, said: "you both are fun and I predict that you will have a great time together." She was right.

A special note of thanks for proofreading is in order to Madeleine Kattan, Lily Kattan, Xinge Ji, Evan Murphy, Shreya Louis, Caroline El Sanadi, Helene Charlotte Wiese Rytgaard, Paul Blanche, Les Dalton, and Antoine Gey.

Michael W Kattan & Thomas A Gerds
September 2020

Terminology

AUC

Area under the receiver operating characteristic curve. Measure of model discriminative ability.

Brier score

Distance between observed event status and predicted risk.

Censored data

Subject is not followed through the entire study period. The event of interest has not yet happened by the end of follow-up.

Competing risks

Event after which the event of interest cannot happen or is not of interest anymore.

Cross-validation

Repeated splitting of a dataset into a learning dataset for model building and a validation dataset for assessment of predictive performance.

Hazard rate

Event probability per time unit: the "speed" of the event of interest.

Hazard ratio

Ratio between two hazard rates.

Hyperparameter/tuning factor

These determine how the modeling algorithm finds the final model.

IPA

Index of Prediction Accuracy. Measure of overall predictive performance relative to a null model.

Modeling algorithm

Computer program that maps a purpose dataset to a risk prediction model.

Null model

Model that ignores predictor variables and predicts an average risk.

Risk prediction model

Computer program that maps patients' characteristics to predicted t-year risk.

Penalty

Hyperparameter used to control overfitting of regression models.

Prediction time horizon

Defines the target of prediction. For example, when set to 5 years, the target is the probability of the event within 5 years.

Predictive performance

Umbrella term for discrimination, calibration, and overall accuracy.

Purpose dataset

Dataset used to build a medical risk prediction model.

Random seed

Control of the random number generator. Potentially, the seed affects machine learning methods and also any form of cross-validation.

Ridge regression

Regression with penalty to shrink regression coefficients.

Restricted cubic spline

Flexible relationship between a continuous predictor variable and the risk of the event.

Risk prediction

Subject-specific probability of the outcome event within the prediction time horizon.

Subject matter expert

This could very well be you.

Target population

Subjects who can use the medical risk prediction model.

Time origin

Start of follow-up and time when the prediction is evaluated.

t-year risk

Probability that the event of interest occurs within time t after the time origin.

Software

The book is illustrated with `R-code`, which is available at

https://github.com/tagteam/MedicalRiskPredictionModels

The repository provides computer-modified versions of data that were kindly provided to us by our collaborators:

- In vitro fertilization study (thanks to Dr. Nina la Cour Freiesleben)

- Oral cancer study (thanks to Dr. Snehal Patel)

- Active surveillance prostate cancer study (thanks to Dr. Kasper Drimer Berg)

1

Why should I care about statistical prediction models?

The backbone of medical decision making is prediction. Clinicians must predict what the patients have, what their outcomes might be, and what might change if treatment is administered. Few things are certain in medicine; most involve probabilities, which must be estimated. Statistical prediction models can help in medical decision making. For example, the comparative effectiveness movement is largely about conveying the probabilities of benefits and harms associated with various alternatives, such as treatments. These predictions facilitate medical decision making and help with the evaluation of medical strategies.

Decision makers, such as patients, need guidance on what options there are and what is likely to happen in the medical future. An analogy between bike riding and life can be used to explain the situation (see Figure 1.1 for a cartoon which illustrates this): the speed of the cyclist on the road corresponds to the hazard rate of the event of interest. The time the cyclist needs to ride from where he is now to a fixed place further down the road corresponds to the absolute risk of the event within a fixed time in the future. Knowing that the speed of one cyclist is 10% higher than that of another cyclist corresponds to knowing that the hazard rate of one patient is 10% higher than that of another patient, i.e., the hazard ratio is 1.1. How much longer the slower cyclist needs to get to the fixed place depends on the distance to this place. Correspondingly, how much more likely the patient with the higher hazard rate is to experience the event of interest depends on the fixed time in the future. In real life, the absolute risk of the event of interest within a fixed time horizon also depends on the hazard rate of the competing risk (such as death without the event).

It is natural to take the viewpoint of the single patient and ask: What does it mean that a risk prediction model performs well? Obviously, a single patient either experiences the event or does not, so a perfect model would have to predict 0% or 100% event probability and get all of those predictions correct. However, when predictions are about the future, such a perfect model does not exist. The reason is that the model can only use information available at the time point when the prediction is given to the patient (called the time origin, the baseline date, or time 0), and things that happen after this time origin are subject to uncertainty. Usually, a meaningful prediction for the

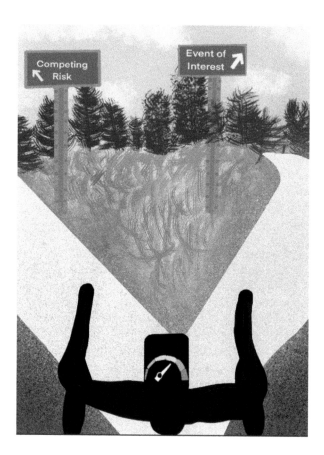

FIGURE 1.1
Eventually, this cyclist will reach either the event of interest or a competing risk. The cyclist considers the current speed and the distance to predict how quickly an event will be reached.

patient also involves a prediction time horizon. Starting at the time origin, a model may predict the probability that the event occurs within the next 5 years. In this example, the prediction time horizon is 5 years. Further, this could be a situation of competing risks, for example, when it may happen that the patient dies without the event before the prediction time horizon. A competing risk is an event after which the event of interest cannot happen or is not of interest anymore for other reasons.

The fundamental principle is the ability to predict the outcome for future patients. Prediction performance measures the distance between the predicted risk and the outcome status (calibration) and the ability to rank patients (discrimination). The yardstick with which all prediction models are assessed is predictive performance. This naturally implies that modeling decisions have a focus on and are guided by prediction performance where possible. This also requires a great deal of care because the predictive performance of a model on the same dataset that was used to build it is not an unbiased indicator of how it would predict on an independent dataset, presumably obtained from the same population. Therefore, it is critical to use modeling tools that do not overfit and will provide unbiased (to the extent possible) assessments of prediction performance.

In this book, we work with two different concepts which can also be combined to make the best possible model. The first is the concept of the *subject matter expert*. With this concept, modeling decisions are based solely on subject matter knowledge and literature but *without* considering the data. The *subject matter expert* could be you or your colleague. The second is the concept of data *cross-validation*, which is the backbone of machine learning [32]. The basic idea is to split the data leaving some for testing. Data-dependent modeling decisions are first learned in one part of the data and then tested in the other part of the data.

1.1 The many uses of prediction models in medicine

Prediction models have many specific uses. The first, and most obvious, is patient counseling. Most patients, when confronted with a worrisome diagnosis, will ask a "Doc, what are my chances?" type of question. Statistical prediction models offer a tailored prediction for this patient, which may serve to counsel him or her. Alternatively, this prediction may suggest to the patient that he or she needs to plan for the future. Another use of prediction models is treatment decision making. A patient would like the treatment that offers the best outcomes. However, these outcomes cannot be known with certainty, and are generally predicted outcomes. Statistical prediction models offer probabilities, usually indicating the likelihood of outcomes, good or bad, within a given prediction time horizon so that the patient (or doctor) can weigh the treatment options. Personal preferences can be combined with statistical predictions to hopefully make the best treatment decision. The third use of prediction models is the selection of patients for clinical trials. Trials of new treatments are generally restricted to patients at high risk of a bad outcome (e.g., disease recurrence) if a standard treatment (alone) is provided. Statistical prediction models, when based on patients who received standard treatment, can be used to identify these high-risk patients so that they may be offered participation in the clinical trial. A fourth use lies in the development of personalized medicine in general, and specifically, the detection of new biomarkers. Individualized predictions based on demographics and conventional markers are compared to those obtained with a statistical model which also includes the values of a new biomarker to hopefully improve predictions.

1.2   The unique messages of this book

1. We devote attention to absolute risks of events occurring between time zero and a fixed prediction time horizon on a continuous probability scale. The probability of survival until a prediction time horizon, say 5 years, is the overwhelmingly popular and most valuable form of statistical prediction modeling. Our concentration on this particular setting allows us to focus on the issues at stake, and as such, make concrete recommendations for the development and assessment of performance.

2. We introduce the concept of visualizing a clinically meaningful change in predicted risks as an aspect of model evaluation. It has always been a problem to judge a prediction model with respect to how well one model predicts relative to another or to no model at all. The existing measures, as a general rule, are not terribly meaningful to the decision maker concerning whether to use the model, which is often decided by the clinician. For example, if a new model has an area under the receiver operating characteristic curve (AUC) that is 0.02 greater than that of the old model, most end users do not know whether this is a large improvement or not. We advance an approach of graphically examining how often the predictions of a new model are changed enough to matter to the end user. This way, we do not simply look at an improvement in predictive accuracy but address whether the change is clinically meaningful.

3. We advocate a machine learning mindset to guide modeling with a focus on predictive performance. For example, ridge regression defines shrinkage in the form of a penalized likelihood; this is a valuable step in the prediction modeling process but is underuti-

lized. While sometimes it will not help much, other times it will. Our cross-validation approach uses the Brier score to choose the penalty parameter, i.e., the amount of shrinkage, this helps to ensure that shrinkage will not hurt the performance of the model. Thus, the shrinkage step often helps some, sometimes helps a lot, and generally will not hurt the performance of the model.

4. For survival endpoints we illustrate the advantage of both the time-dependent Brier score and the time-dependent AUC over the more commonly used concordance index. This is important due to the overwhelming popularity of the concordance index. However, we show that these other approaches, time-dependent Brier score and time-dependent AUC, offer important advantages in most prediction model settings because the endpoint is typically the probability of survival beyond a prediction time horizon. The concordance index for survival data does not evaluate this target directly.

5. We try to create the best of both worlds when choosing between traditional statistical techniques and newer machine learning approaches. First, we apply the machine learning mindset to improve standard regression models by using cross validation extensively and focusing on predictive accuracy. We compare machine learning models with standard regression models. Sometimes, we even combine the two approaches, as is done in a super learner.

6. We provide thorough instruction on the development and evaluation of prediction models in the presence of competing risks. This is noteworthy since a model that ignores competing risks can be misleading, and the methods for developing and validating models that properly account for competing risks are not well disseminated. Ignoring the presence of competing risks creates a hypothetical world where the competing risk has been removed. For example, ignoring the competing risk of death creates a hypothetical world where patients cannot die. This setup makes for a very artificial prediction.

7. We argue that the validation of a prediction model, in isolation from other prediction models, is not terribly useful. It makes much more sense to compare rival models on a dataset that was not used to build either rival model (sometimes called a "neutral" dataset). One such benchmark, which we illustrate, is the null model, which any model should outperform. Simply examining the performance of a single model on one or more datasets does not add too much knowledge unless the model performs horribly.

8. We describe several variations of model validation analysis. *To validate* means to test the performance of a risk prediction model in new data. To do this correctly, in an unbiased fashion, repeated splitting of the purpose dataset into learning and validation is needed. This

is called cross validation. A single split of the dataset into one learning dataset and one validation dataset has the huge drawback that results depend on *how* the data were split. Structural splits using, e.g., calendar time or medical center, are innocent, but results of a single *random split* of the purpose dataset depend crucially on the random seed; and important medical decisions should never depend on the lucky number of the analyst. We also point out that creating a single split of the purpose dataset does not create an "external" validation dataset, but it surely reduces the amount of data available to build the final risk prediction model. Repeated model building in many learning datasets, on the other hand, requires a pre-specified computer program called the *modeling algorithm*. The great advantage of repeated data splitting is that the final risk prediction model is obtained by applying the modeling algorithm to the full dataset. With many human decisions made by the analyst that are motivated by looking closer at the data, it can be hard to prespecify and implement all steps of modeling in a computer program. In this case, a single split of the data is still better than simply testing the model on the exact same data used to build the model. However, leaving part of the data aside for validation, in some sense, wastes those data since they do not contribute to the model-building process, but some journals (e.g., Journal of Clinical Oncology) give lower priority to studies that do not leave data out. So, despite efficiency concerns, political reasons may dictate that a single-split analysis should be performed. The strongest form of validation of a risk prediction model is a prospective study where patients are randomized to either use or not use the prediction model, and data are collected on clinical outcomes, as well as on patient satisfaction.

1.3   Prognostic factor modeling philosophy

Within the field of statistical prediction model development, there are two competing schools of thought. The argument is mostly philosophical, but there is a debate between theory-driven and data-driven variable selection. The theory-driven camp argues that subject matter experts are the best way to identify predictors that belong or do not belong in a statistical prediction model. They feel that this yields many benefits, most importantly higher likelihood of physician buy-in. At the end of the day, the decision to use a medical statistical prediction model rests with the physician: She or he must believe in the model, or it will not get used. Therefore, including the variables that a physician believes should be included goes a long way toward model dissemination and uptake. Non-experts who are fishing in available data may select nonsensical variables that will make the model look strange to the physician, or they may select predictor variables that are not actually available at the time the model needs to be executed. Problems like these are avoided when relying upon the expert to specify how he or she thinks the predictor variables play into the outcome.

On the other hand, restricting variable selection to the subject matter expert, in the theory-driven approach, is limiting. One cannot stumble upon the previously unknown predictor that is actually beneficial to the model. Moreover, one cannot find the statistical interaction that was not specified by the subject matter expert. Thus, the data-driven approach has more flexibility in the models that are examined. The data-driven approach heavily relies on cross validation and cross fitting. This requires that all modeling steps are available in the form of computer code and can be applied to fit a model in each fold of the data. Instead of pre-specifying a single regression model, the data-driven approach selects a library of regression models and other prediction modeling algorithms. Then, one either chooses the model which has the highest cross validated performance, or one constructs the final model by weighing the individual models in a clever way using the best of each model to construct a super learner.

1.4 The rest of this book

Now the stage has been set. The philosophy behind and rationale for building and evaluating statistical prediction models is behind us. The rest of this book deals with how to do this and what you need to know to be successful.

2

I am going to make a prediction model. What do I need to know?

This chapter contains essential background reading that any serious modeler needs to know. Some of this is terminology, and some of this is philosophy.

2.1 Prediction model framework

2.1.1 Target population

The target population consists of all subjects who would be eligible to use the model. It is conveniently defined by a series of inclusion and exclusion criteria that are often displayed in the form of a flow diagram.

2.1.2 The time origin

The framework for a risk prediction model starts by defining a common time origin for all subjects in a well-defined population. This is typically a time point at which the clinical setting is augmented by new information, such as a new diagnosis, a new measurement of a biomarker, or the start of treatment. The time origin also defines when the prediction can be interpreted by a new patient. In some settings, the time origin is defined directly by the purpose. For example, the date of diagnosis with cancer or the date of the start of treatment are natural time origins for cancer patients. In other settings, the time origin is less clearly defined. For example, when the aim is to predict the risk of cardiovascular disease in the general population, there is not an obvious time origin. It is then an essential part of the prediction modeling task to define the time origin.

2.1.3 The event of interest

In a broad sense, the event of interest is the onset of a new medical condition in a single person/patient. It is the object of the prediction task and naturally defined by the subject matter context. For example, the event of interest can be a stroke. In some settings, there are multiple events that need to be predicted.

For example, a patient who starts blood-thinning therapy, in addition to a prediction of the risk of stroke, should be interested in a prediction of the risk of major bleeding. In cases with competing risks, there are several alternative options to define the event of interest (see Section 2.4.6). For some medical conditions, it is difficult to determine the exact date of onset. Diabetes is an example. Here, either the date of the first measurement of the blood marker A1C above a threshold or the date of the start of anti-diabetic medicine is used as a proxy for the onset of diabetes. Thus, to be precise, the event which is predictable based on data is not *diabetes* but *diagnosis of diabetes*.

2.1.4   The prediction time horizon and follow-up

The prediction time horizon is any time point after the time origin.

> *The special case where the aim is to predict/diagnose the patient's current status is included by setting the prediction time horizon equal to the time origin.*

The prediction time horizon should be chosen such that it is of subject matter interest to predict the probability that the event occurs in the time period between the time origin and the prediction time horizon. For the patients whose data are included in the training dataset, it should be known or at least known up to certain limitations, whether or not the event has occurred between the time origin and the prediction time horizon. Limitations are either related to difficulties in measuring the event or to early end of follow up. To discuss an example of the latter, suppose the prediction time horizon is set 5 years after the time origin. For patients who experience the event of interest within their individual follow-up period, the event status at 5 years is known (uncensored). For a patient whose individual follow-up period ends before the prediction time horizon, the event status at the prediction time horizon is unknown (right-censored). For patients who die event-free (or experience any other competing risk) before the prediction time horizon, the event status at the prediction time horizon is also known: "no event" (Figure 2.1).

Soft and surrogate endpoints, such as recurrence of cancer, are often difficult to measure because they require that the patient is examined by an expert and the result thus depends on both the diagnostic tool and the schedule of follow-up examinations. It is therefore necessary to describe the exact construction of the event time (or the event status at the prediction time horizon) which is to be used as the "outcome" in the purpose dataset (Section 2.4.1). It is sometimes useful to study multiple prediction time horizons, but this should be motivated by the application at hand (beware of cherry-picking).

It should also be reported what treatments patients received during the follow-up period prior to the event of interest (or competing risk). Although such information is not useful as a predictor or the outcome variable, it is needed to ensure generalizability of the model to future settings.

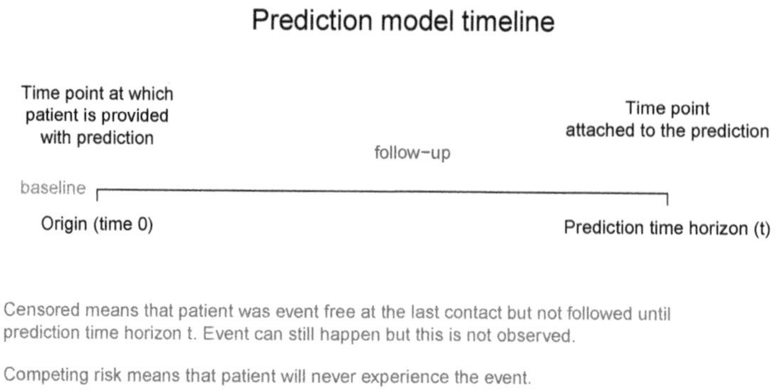

Prediction model timeline

Time point at which
patient is provided
with prediction

Time point
attached to the prediction

follow−up

baseline

Origin (time 0)

Prediction time horizon (t)

Censored means that patient was event free at the last contact but not followed until
prediction time horizon t. Event can still happen but this is not observed.

Competing risk means that patient will never experience the event.

FIGURE 2.1
Illustration of prediction model framework.

2.1.5   Landmarking

It is possible and sometimes useful to work with multiple time origins. These
time points are then called landmark times and correspondingly the statistical
analyses are called landmark analyses [178, 177]. Note that at each landmark
time point, the purpose dataset (Section 2.4.1) is different; it contains only
the data of those patients who, in addition to satisfying baseline inclusion/ex-
clusion criteria, are alive and event-free at the landmark time point. In this
way, a series of prediction models can be obtained which can be used to monitor patients based on dynamic updates of the predictions. At each landmark,
the predicted risk still corresponds to a defined prediction time horizon. It is
possible to update predictor variables that have changed value between the
baseline date and the landmark date (Sections 6.4.2 and 7.7).

2.1.6   Risks and risk predictions

A risk is the probability that an adverse event happens. A chance is the
probability that a positive event happens. A survival chance is the probability
that an adverse event does not happen. In the absence of competing risks (see
Sections 2.1.4 and 2.4.6), the risk of the adverse event can be calculated by
subtracting the corresponding survival chance from 100%. In the presence of
a competing risk, this relationship is generally lost (Section 2.7.5).

   Risks are tied to and interpreted with respect to a given time period in
which the event can happen to an individual (Figure 2.1). A risk prediction is
an estimate of the risk based on a purpose dataset (see Section 2.4.1) which
contains information from previous patients. Risk predictions are personal
statistics, tailored to the patient based on individual characteristics.

2.1.7 Classification of risk

A very common form of medical risk dissemination is in terms of risk groups. Examples are cancer staging systems and the Charlson comorbidity index. In this book we prefer to work with predictions in terms of probabilities. The predicted risk p is the probability that the event of interest happens to a given subject. We should note that based on a probabilistic prediction, risk groups can be generated as follows. Any single fixed threshold value c between 0 and 1 transforms predicted risks p into predicted class (yes vs. no). Since the observed is also yes vs. no, one can cross classify the observations by both predicted and observed. This defines a so-called confusion matrix:

Predicted class	Event	No event
$p > c$	Number of correct positives	Number of false positives
$p \leq c$	Number of false negatives	Number of correct negatives

This is a cross table with the observed outcome on one dimension and predicted class on the other dimension. It is then possible to define sensitivity, specificity, negative and positive predictive value, etc., but the results depend on the value c, and there is no good reason to choose $c = 50\%$.

By varying the threshold c we can actually have a receiver operating characteristic curve (ROC) curve [65] (see also Chapter 5) and could in principle have a precision-recall curve [148]. We could also discuss the Youden index, the Matthew correlation coefficient and many other "optimal" threshold values. A technical issue here is that the statistical uncertainty about the actual value of any "optimal" threshold found in a dataset is generally large. More problematic is the following argument. First, note that we would lose information when we transform the predicted risk into a predicted class. If indeed the aim would be to decide about medical intervention directly by choosing a fixed threshold for the predicted risk for all patients, then we would need to integrate this into all steps of modeling where now the target would not be to predict the risk but to predict the class. Ideally, we would guide the search for the best risk classifier (a model which assigns class membership) by costs and benefits of the corresponding medical decision (see also Section 2.2.7).

But, in this book, we generally do not take the situation so far as to evaluate medical decisions that are directly read off the result of a statistical risk prediction model. The main reason is that in most clinical settings the prediction of the model is used to inform the clinician and the patient, but the final decision about actual medical intervention is the responsibility of the clinician and the patient (see also Section 9.1). In this book, the outcome of the model is a predicted risk and not a predicted class.

2.1.8 Predictor variables

A predictor is a variable that is both known at the time origin (or landmark time point) and used for calculating the predicted risks. A predictor variable can simply be a characteristic of the patient such as the current age, the gender, or whether the patient has diabetes (see Section 3.4). It can also be a measurement of a biomarker such as obtained with a blood test or a derived variable (Section 3.4.3). Predictors are the essential part of the formula which makes the prediction, and predictors are weighted, somehow, by the statistical model for predicting personalized risks (Chapter 4).

2.1.9 Checklist

Checklist for a prediction model framework

- Target population: Describe who would be eligible to use the model and whatever inclusion/exclusion criteria should be applied.

- Time origin: Describe the baseline or prognostic time zero, i.e., at which time the event prediction will be calculated in future patients.

- Target of prediction: Describe the event of interest (e.g., all-cause death, disease-specific death, onset or recurrence of disease).

- Competing risks: Describe events after which the event of interest cannot occur (e.g., death) or is not of interest any longer (e.g., transplant).

- Prediction time horizon: How far in time from the time origin (e.g., 10-year survival probability) the prediction is projected.

- Predictor variables: List the predictors measured at baseline and how they were measured.

2.2 Prediction performance

The measurement of the performance of a risk prediction model is a complex subject. The ultimate performance parameter would be a measure of the impact of the model, for example, the number of lives which can be improved when the prediction model is applied. However, this is difficult to quantify in most cases. Less ambitious parameters that characterize the prediction performance of a model include accuracy, calibration, and discrimination. At this stage, it is important to recognize that there is not a single measure of performance by means of which risk prediction models can be assessed and compared. David Hand stated this fact in the following way [85]. *"It would be incorrect to assert that any one of these ways was 'wrong' and others 'right' –*

they merely measure different things – but, in general, one should match one's measure of performance to what one is trying to achieve."

2.2.1 Proper scoring rules

A scoring rule compares the observed outcomes to the predicted risks. Here, the observed outcome is a binary variable (at the prediction time horizon) which takes the value 1 or 100% for subjects who experienced the event and the value 0 for subjects who did not. On the other hand, the predicted risks of the event of interest are values between 0 and 100%. It is better when the individual predicted risks are closer to the observed outcome status at the prediction time horizon. When measuring performance as an error, the difference between observed and predicted, a low average score is desirable, the lower, the better.

Scoring rules are useful to compare rival risk prediction models. For this the scoring rule should be proper, i.e., have propriety. In order to understand what this implies, consider a group of experts and a sample of subjects. Each expert provides a predicted risk for each subject. Suppose further that the experts are rivals, eager to provide the best prediction as if this were a betting game. The scoring rule is used to find the winner. The scoring rule is proper if (in the long run) no expert can win over the biological model that generates the data, i.e., over the true event probability. More specifically the scoring rule is called strictly proper if there is no shared first place, i.e., any expert's prediction model cannot score equally well (in the long run) if it deviates from the data-generating model. Seminal work by Leonard Savage [158] shows that the main proper scoring rules for probabilistic predictions (i.e., predictions formulated as probability of the event) are the Brier score, which computes the square of the difference between observed status and the predicted risk, and the logarithmic score. It is interesting to note that the absolute loss defined by the absolute distance between the predicted risk and the observed status is not a proper scoring rule.

We do not consider the logarithmic score in this book because it yields an infinite value when some predicted risks are exactly zero or exactly one. However, the logarithmic scoring rule is closely related to the log likelihood used as an optimization criterion, and it can very well be used to evaluate risk predictions, where it will give more reward to extreme predictions that are correct.

Why is the propriety of the scoring rule so utterly important? To see this, consider a situation where an improper scoring rule is used to find the best prediction model. Then it may happen that one of the experts has found the best risk prediction model for the target population, but another expert is winning the competition with an inferior model. With an improper scoring rule, it would be possible to show that adding a random noise variable to a logistic regression model is improving the prediction performance [141]. It would also be possible to show that any risk prediction model can be "improved" by making its predictions systematically more extreme [98]. That is why one should never use improper scoring rules.

When we search for the best risk prediction model, we should always remember that two rival models with similar average performance scores in a sample from the target population can predict very different risks to the same individuals. Therefore, it becomes important to look closely at the individual predicted probabilities.

2.2.2   Calibration

Suppose the model predicts that an event will occur for a patient with a probability of 12%. The patient will expect to be event-free since this probability is much larger (88%). If it turns out that the event did not occur, then one could argue that the model did well for this patient. On the other hand, if the event occurs, then one could argue that he/she was one of the 12%. We call a predicted risk of x% *reliable* if it can be expected that the event will occur to x out of 100 patients who all received a predicted risk of x%. A model is well *calibrated* in a given population if the risk predictions given to all subjects in the population are *reliable*.

Calibration of the prediction model is important for the patient, for patient counseling and medical decision making, and in particular personalized medicine. If a patient is told that he has an 80% chance of an outcome, he would like to be assured that if there were 100 patients just like him, 80 would experience the event. This is calibration. More specifically, this is called calibration in the small. Calibration in the large refers to a comparison of the average prediction in the group of all patients (one value) with the average observed outcome (one value). Calibration in the large will typically be good for a model that has good calibration in the small. However, what matters for the individual patient and for the purpose of making a risk prediction model is calibration in the small.

2.2.3   Discrimination

Discrimination evaluates a specific aspect of a model's predictive performance, namely, its ability to rank subjects according to the risk of an event. Thus, a model that predicts the same value for all patients has zero ability to discriminate. We say that a model *discriminates* well when, for any two patients where one has the event and the other does not, the one with the event received the higher predicted risk from the model. Since discrimination is the ability of a model to rank patients, high discrimination is nice to have, but it is not sufficient to indicate that the risk prediction model has value. The reason for this is that a well-discriminating model may have poor calibration.

The main measure for risk discrimination is the area under the receiver operating characteristic curve (AUC). It is sometimes called the AUROC, or the c-statistic, or the concordance index. For time-to-event outcomes we consider the time-dependent AUC (Chapter 5). In Chapter 9 we explain why the time-dependent AUC [92] is better suited for our prediction model framework than the popular Harrell's c-index [88] and variants thereof. Note further that the Gini index, which is popular in economics and machine learning, is simply calculated as $2 * \text{AUC} - 1$.

2.2.4 Explained variation

Explained variation is a term that is used to describe how much of the variation of the outcome can be explained by the predictor variables, more precisely by a model that uses the predictor variables. The classical measure of explained variation is R^2. In the linear regression model setting, it is defined as the complement to 100% of the residual sum of squares of the model divided by the total sum of squares. The total sum of squares is obtained based on the residuals of the null model, which ignores all covariates and simply predicts the average outcome for all subjects. In order to extend this definition to models for the binary outcome and censored survival outcomes, many alternative definitions of explained variation and estimators have been derived, see for example [151].

In this book, we restrict the focus to explained variation, defined in the same way as R^2 for the linear model, where we use the Brier scores to define patient-specific residuals. That is, instead of squaring the difference between a continuous outcome and its prediction, we square the difference between a binary outcome (event yes/no at the prediction time horizon) and the predicted risk. Note that this assumes the outcome event is coded as 1, in the same direction as the predicted risk. This type of measure has been proposed by many, e.g., [118, 172] and it can be estimated based on censored data [82]. Moreover, the measure extends to competing risks. We call this measure the Index of Prediction Accuracy (IPA) [115] (Section 5.5).

2.2.5 Variability and uncertainty

From a practical viewpoint, the predicted probability sufficiently conveys the extent of uncertainty. For example, a value of 50% is much more uncertain than a value of 2% or 98%. However, there are different components in the uncertainty and variability in a risk prediction coming from a statistical model. Uncertainty about the predicted risk is related to the amount of data in the purpose dataset. The higher the sample size, the more can be learned from the data and hence the lower the uncertainty. Clearly, the nature of the modeling algorithm used also plays a role. Hence, the interpretation of the predicted risk should change whether it is the result of a complex machine learning algorithm applied to a small purpose dataset or the result of a logistic regression model with pre-specified variables applied to a large purpose dataset. Independent of the modeling algorithm it may happen that subjects with extreme values of the predictor variables are more likely to experience higher uncertainty in their predictions than are subjects with common predictor values [76]. However, not much can be done about this, other than to potentially limit the predictions to those with more central values, but this is a subject matter judgment call.

Intuitively one might think that a confidence interval around the prediction would help convey the uncertainty of the prediction. However, confidence intervals for predicted probabilities are quite tricky to interpret and as such have a limited role in conveying uncertainty. However, for the sake of interpretability, in the often-difficult situation for the patient, it is generally important that small perturbations of the data lead to unimportant changes in the risk predictions. In other words, a modeling algorithm should be rejected if it is unstable in the sense that adding or removing one or a few patients from the purpose dataset generates gross changes in the risk predictions of a subgroup of the patients. As an alternative to the confidence interval, it is often useful to see how much the predicted risk of single individuals change under perturbation of the purpose dataset, for example, when 10% of the data are removed and the model is re-fitted.

2.2.6   The interpretation is relative

Some say an AUC around 75% is good and 85% is very good, etc. We strongly discourage this practice (see Figure 5.5). The caveat with such a situation-free interpretation is that the performance of the model depends on the situation, here in particular on the distribution of the risk factors in the target population. For example, a risk prediction model for which age is an important variable will have a higher AUC in a population where the subjects have different ages than in a population where the subjects are similar with respect to age.

Generally, the absolute values of the Brier score, IPA, and AUC metrics cannot be compared across different fields of application or datasets because these metrics depend on the distributions of the predictor variable values. In other words, when the case-mix of patients is different in a location, this will affect the performance metrics of a risk prediction model. Instead, we compare these performance metrics to their benchmark values (Chapter 5), and we compare rival models (Chapter 6).

2.2.7   Utility

The utility of a prediction model usually refers to an aspect of patient preferences, and it is always tied to some form of decision about an intervention, such as "to treat" or "not to treat." Thus, the utility of a prediction model will often refer to its value in medical decision making. A risk prediction model can be accurate but be of little utility if it does not help facilitate a decision. When a prediction model is implemented and it causes many meaningful changes in the risk estimation, it can be of great utility assuming the decisions it affects lead to good choices. However, it is generally difficult to measure the utility of a model. One reason is that one needs to quantify the costs and benefits of the different interventions on some scale. Another reason is that in most clinical settings the decision about intervention is not only based on the result of the model, but influenced by the responsible clinician and the preferences of the patient. Note that the most valid way to test the utility of a prediction model is to randomize patients to receive the predictions from the model or not, and then observing later patient outcomes.

2.2.8   Average versus subgroups

Another challenge when the focus of modeling is to predict the individual outcome is that results have to be meaningful for individuals and accurate not just on average. For example, a new model may be seen to predict better on average in a given population than the conventional model, but there may still exist a subgroup of patients who are better off with the conventional model. Thus, also the performance of a statistical prediction model should be measured on the individual level to the extent possible, for example in subgroups.

2.3   Study design

2.3.1   Study design and sources of information

In order to make a prediction model, you need individual person-level data. In the ideal case, these are extracted from a cohort database with a well-defined start of follow-up. Case-control data are insufficient for prediction model building; you will need additional information to utilize data from the case-control study in a prediction model [18]. Data from a randomized clinical trial can be used to build a prediction model; however, some practical rules need to be obeyed. One is that predictions can only be interpreted in connection with one of the treatments of the trial. In other words, it is generally assumed that the patient follows a certain treatment strategy when interpreting the predicted risk of the event. Another is that the patient seeking advice from such a model needs to satisfy the inclusion and exclusion criteria of the trial in order to be applicable for the prediction model.

Particular characteristics of the dataset will dictate whether you can actually build a prediction model from them and how to build the prediction model. For example, it is going to make things much easier if the data were collected in a manner similar to the setting in which you would like the prediction model deployed. Say a model predicts the 5-year risk of death following a surgical procedure. Does the dataset contain all patients who received this surgical procedure over a particular time frame? And were they all followed for 5 years? If patients were excluded from the purpose dataset for outcome-related reason, serious ramifications for the prediction model can result.

2.3.2   Cohort

Cohort studies work best for prediction model development. A cohort is often a sample of generally consecutive patients enrolled over time. They are not selected based on their outcome. All patients who meet baseline inclusion and exclusion criteria are included in the target population. Patients in a cohort will often have varying lengths of follow-up. Cohort studies are typically larger in size with a more diverse patient mix than prospectively planned studies but tend to have data collection errors and missing values. It is thus difficult to make a definitive statement as to which type of data is preferred. One point is clear: it should not be assumed that prediction models developed from randomized clinical trials are "correct" and models developed from cohorts in research databases are "wrong." Models need to be evaluated and compared to determine accuracy, and we address this further in Chapters 5 and 6.

2.3.3   Multi-center study

A multi-center study can, in principle, be used as the basis of a prediction model. However, it is not self-evident that predictions improve when data from centers are combined for modeling. In this case, it is particularly important to carefully check the calibration of the model's predictions in centers that were not part of the modeling. Usually it is desired that the model be applicable to centers beyond those that contributed data, so it is important that the predictions do not depend on the center. If such dependence occurs, it is not straightforward to remedy by introducing a random effect to describe heterogeneity between centers or by treating the center as a characteristic of the subjects, and may, in fact, not always be achievable (Section 7.1).

2.3.4   Randomized clinical trial

Data from randomized clinical trials offer advantages for model building. These data are prospectively and carefully collected. Errors and missing values are thus minimized. However, strong selection criteria are applied. As a result, prediction models emanating from randomized clinical trial data tend to have a narrow focus in terms of patients who can have predictions obtained. These studies are like cohorts, in that consecutive patients are enrolled. However, in a randomized clinical trial, the treatment is assigned randomly. With a cohort, the treatment is chosen by the doctor and patient.

The strongest form of validation of a risk prediction model is a prospective study where patients are randomized to use or not use the prediction model, and data are collected on clinical outcomes, as well as on patient satisfaction. The drawback here is that prospective validation will require at least as long as the prediction horizon of the model before it can be performed (e.g., prospectively validating a 5-year prediction model will take over 5 years to do). By that time, the prediction model may be obsolete, so demanding that a prediction model be prospectively validated is typically being overly cautious because it denies future patients (e.g., those diagnosed within the next 5 years) the use of a potentially better prediction model.

2.3.5 Case-control

Case-control designs complicate prediction model building, especially when the outcome is a time-to-event variable (where censoring occurs). However, nested case-control studies can be performed [156]. Case-control studies are not nearly as useful for prediction model building because patients have been selected based on their observed outcomes. This makes it more difficult to assess the probabilities of outcomes because the overall rate of outcomes has been disturbed by the patient selection process. Benichou and Gail [18] discussed inference methods for risk predictions derived from a case-control study.

2.3.6 Given treatment and treatment options

In many applications, the patients who end up in the purpose dataset were treated according to some guidelines. The aim of the prediction model could be to change the guidelines. The holy grail of prediction model evaluation is the setting where you can randomize patients to either receipt of prediction from the model or standard of care.

More generally, predictions associated with the treatment options are the basis of the decision-making process, which will typically also involve consideration of side effects and quality of life. Ideally, a future patient will be counseled by providing two (or more) predictions, one for each treatment. With comparative effectiveness tables, these predictions are tailored to the individual patient at hand, unlike the common group-level (or even risk-group-based) treatment recommendations. This topic is discussed further in Section 7.2.

2.3.7 Sample size calculation

Researchers will frequently ask about the (minimum) sample size required to build a prediction model. It is useful to plan a study that aims to build a risk prediction model. However, as with any other sample size and power calculation problem, the nature of the specific target parameter needs to be taken into account. When each subject in the population receives a different predicted risk from the model, the target of the prediction model is not a single hypothesis test for which standard power calculations apply. Thus, without additional quantification of the benefits and harms, one may choose to focus on population average prediction performance as measured by suitable metrics (Chapter 5). The specific aim could be to plan a validation study for an existing risk prediction model, or to identify new predictive markers which improve the performance of an existing risk prediction model, or to develop a new risk prediction model. The reason the sample size calculation for these questions is complex is that the performance of the statistical prediction model is affected by many things, including:

1. sample size [more is better];

2. data quality [less measurement error and fewer missing values are better];

3. predictors [collecting important predictors obviously helps];

4. statistical modeling approach [sound methods and tuning via cross-validation helps].

Hence, an appropriate setup for a sample size calculation needs to be provided with information regarding data quality, predictors, and the statistical modeling approach. Existing research on this subject is typically focused on a fully specified regression model, for example, by specifying the number of events needed per predictor variable [41]. However, rules of thumb (e.g., 10 events per model degree of freedom, discussed in Section 9.2) and other ad hoc formulas are too simple, because they do not address the process of finding the best prediction model, where one, for example, learns which predictor variables should be included and how. Our recommendation is that the best approach to power and sample size calculation is to simulate data with the computer using different sample sizes and some criterion for the desired population average prediction performance. Ideally, the simulated data are like the real data and all data-dependent steps of modeling are applied in order to determine the appropriate sample size. However, simulating data for the purposes of sample size determination are beyond the scope of this book.

2.4   Data

2.4.1   Purpose dataset

At the time origin, all patients who are alive and event-free at that time point (who also satisfy additional inclusion/exclusion criteria of the target population) are included in the purpose dataset. The purpose dataset is the dataset completely ready for prediction modeling. The covariates to be used as predictors have been properly formatted, with sparse predictor variable values collapsed, if there were any. For our purposes, the outcome variable is either a single binary variable or the pair of variables featuring the time to the event and the event indicator. In most cases, these are consecutively identified subjects over a particular time frame (i.e., between two calendar dates, which should be stated) after inclusion and exclusion criteria (which also should be stated) have been applied. In the time-to-event setting, the event indicator is usually coded such that 0 means no event, 1 means event, and when there are competing risks they are coded as 2.

2.4.2 Data dictionary

The data dictionary is a separate file which contains details for each variable in the purpose dataset. These details include units of measurement (e.g., 0 = female, 1 = male, age in years), reasons for missing values and measurement error, and information on how each variable was measured (e.g., particular assay, when the patient was fasting, using a particular device). The main reason for the data dictionary is to guide the modeling. Here it can sometimes be useful to note the biologically plausible range of a variable, and also the biologically expected direction of the effect on the outcome for a variable, e.g., "females have lower risk." One other reason for the data dictionary is to allow others to derive a validation dataset in the same manner as was used for the construction of the development dataset. Moreover, the data dictionary allows the clinician to select the correct values when running the prediction model.

2.4.3 Measurement error

The values of a predictor variable may depend on the way it is measured and generally be subject to measurement error. The total amount of measurement error will often be a composition of several effects. For example, the measurement of a subject's blood pressure will often depend on who performs the measurement (white coat hypertension), the actual apparatus, and whether the subject is sitting or standing during the measurement. Another example is when predictor variables are defined based on a diagnostic imaging procedure such as CT scanning that requires that an expert reads the value. The severity of the resulting measurement error is often assessed by inter-rater agreement.

No matter where it is coming from, measurement error can potentially dilute the usefulness of a risk prediction model. To minimize the risk of a wrong conclusion, where appropriate, one should provide instructions on how to measure the predictor variables and any information about expected measurement error along with the risk prediction model.

2.4.4 Missing values

The dataset used for building the prediction model may contain predictors with missing values. Missing data often generate non-trivial challenges that the modeler cannot ignore. In order to reduce bias during modeling, the most important question is why the data are missing. Thus, it is highly recommended that data collection forms prohibit completion when there are missing values if possible, and in any case, record and distinguish reasons for missing values separately for each predictor variable.

In order to avoid bias in conclusions of any subsequent statistical analysis, it is necessary to know as much as possible about the reasons why a value of a variable can be missing. For example, a missing result of an electrocardiogram has a different interpretation when it is missing because the patient was too weak to perform the test as compared to when it is missing because the measurement device was out of order that day. The crucial difference is that in the latter case the reason is independent of the status of the patient. It should be described how missing data were dealt with (see Section 7.5).

2.4.5   Censored data

A common behavior is that patients with short follow-up are excluded from the dataset. This is almost never the right thing to do, as intuitive as it may seem. Excluding them results in bias.

Outcome at the prediction time horizon can be unknown (censored) for some subjects in the dataset. For example, this would be the case for all subjects who were not followed until the prediction time horizon and who were free of any event by the end of their individual follow-up period (date of last contact or date of last examination). In either case, data from patients with a censored outcome cannot be ignored and need to enter the model-building process somehow. However, by choosing a prediction time horizon closer to the time origin, generally fewer subjects are censored due to short follow-up. Figure 2.2 illustrates this. At the 5-year prediction time horizon, only patient 5 is censored. At the 10-year prediction time horizon, patients 5 and 6 are censored.

In order to assess the accuracy of the prediction model, we need to know the outcome status of the patients in the test set. In many applications, the status depends on time. For example, if a patient has relapsed after 3 years and 4 months, then the 3-year status is negative, meaning *event-free*, but the 5-year status is positive. Even if we fix the prediction time horizon to be 3 years, unequal follow-up of the test sample patients requires special care. Patients not followed until the prediction time horizon have unknown status at the prediction time horizon and are considered censored.

In many applications, specific estimation techniques are needed to take care of bias due to sampling or due to missing or censored data (Chapters 5 and 7). This depends on the study design and the way data are collected.

2.4.6   Competing risks

Patients may experience a competing risk. A competing risk is any event after which the event of interest either cannot happen anymore or is not of interest anymore. A typical example of the former is death from other causes, after

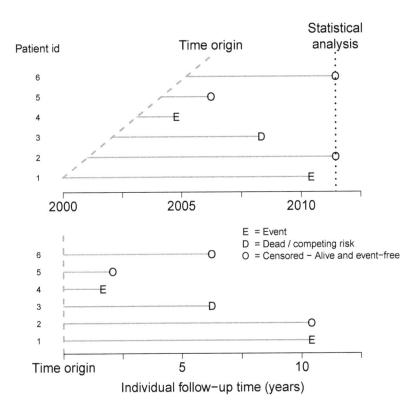

FIGURE 2.2
Illustration of six patients' individual follow-up in a prediction model framework. The upper panel shows how the data are collected in calendar time. The lower panel shows the right-censored time-to-event data. The follow-up of patients 2 and 6 ends at the date of statistical analysis. Patient 5 is lost to follow-up.

which disease recurrence/progression cannot happen anymore (Figure 2.3). An example of the latter is when the event of interest is death due to liver disease and the patient receives a liver transplant.

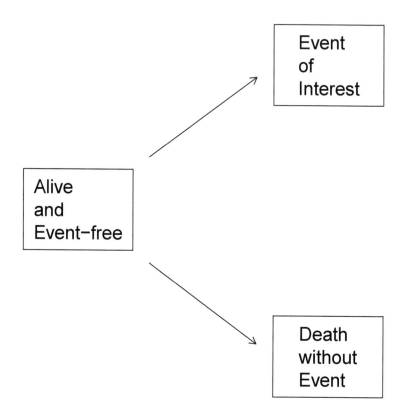

FIGURE 2.3
Competing risk model. At any time, each subject is in one of the three states.

The typical mistake here is to consider that the competing risk (such as death from unrelated causes) is the same as censoring (end of follow-up alive and event-free before the prediction horizon). However, the distinction is important, as bias will result if the competing-risk patients are censored at the time of the competing event. The reason for this lies in the fact that a patient who is lost to follow-up could, with further follow-up, develop the event of interest. But the patient who experiences the competing risk, even with further follow-up, will never develop the event of interest – we know for sure that this patient is a true negative, so he is fully informative, not just partially informative (as is the case with a censored patient). See also Section 2.7.4.

Competing risks will always alter the definition of the event of interest.

For example, instead of the event "kidney failure," we study the event "kidney failure without kidney transplant" when kidney transplant is a competing risk. And often, several definitions make sense in the same setting. For example, consider a study that aims to predict the event "stroke". One can be interested in the event "fatal or non-fatal stroke" with non-stroke-related death being the competing risk. One can also be interested in the event "stroke or death due to cardiovascular causes" with death due to non-cardiovascular causes being the competing risk. Finally, one can define the event "stroke or all-cause death" now without competing risks, and such that the predicted event probability can be interpreted as (one minus) the stroke-free survival probability.

Another interesting situation occurs when disease relapse is the event of interest, and death without relapse is the competing risk. Often, disease relapse must be measured clinically and as such, only "occurs" at the time of a clinic visit. Thus, death in the apparent absence of relapse may have been preceded by relapse, yet this is unknown (i.e., the patient may have an undetected relapse at the time of death). A complex statistical model is needed to describe and analyze the risk of relapse without apparent bias in this setting due to the *interval-censored* nature of the data [173].

Competing risks can generally not be ignored when the aim is patient counseling. In some cases, one would need to consider both the predicted risk of the event of interest and also the predicted risk of the competing event in order to inform the patient about the medical future.

2.5 Modeling

2.5.1 Risk prediction model

A risk prediction model is a tool that, when provided with the predictor values of a new patient, returns a predicted probability. This probability is defined by the prediction model framework (see Section 2.1). To illustrate a completely specified prediction model framework, consider patients with congenital heart disease. Time zero is set at the date of surgery for congenital heart disease. The event of interest is fatal or non-fatal cardiovascular disease and the time horizon is set at 5 years. A risk prediction model thus predicts the 5-year risk of (fatal or non-fatal) cardiovascular disease for all patients who undergo surgery for congenital heart disease.

A risk prediction model can be thought of as a black box where patient characteristics enter one side and a risk prediction comes out on the other side (Figure 2.4). By risk prediction model, we do not necessarily mean a presumed mathematical construct. For example, one can use a random forest model which makes no a priori assumptions, and only learns from the data. Figure 2.5 illustrates the making of a risk prediction model based on a dataset.

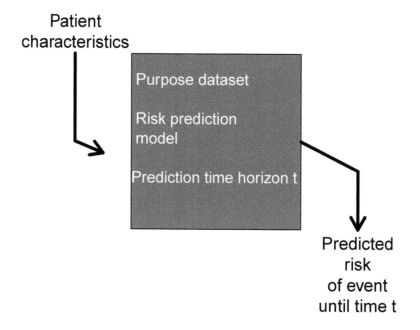

FIGURE 2.4
Illustration of how a risk prediction model works. The data of the new patient enters on one side, the predicted risk comes out on the other side. Inside the box, the model summarizes what happened to earlier patients whose data are stored in the dataset.

We use the term "model" to describe the way we choose to represent the observed data in such a way that is amenable to produce predictions. An analyst whose primary goal is to make predictions, fundamentally, should be agnostic with respect to the mathematical model used for prediction. The primary concern in this respect is prediction performance. Whatever approach can produce the most accurate predictions for future patients should be used. Having said this, most analysts have preferences as to how models should be developed and can point to abundant literature comparing or defending particular methods. Nevertheless, one may argue that accuracy trumps style, and a more accurate prediction model, even when constructed in an unconventional manner, is preferred. However, there are exceptions to this rule, and when using unconventional methods to construct a risk prediction model it is very important to not only look at prediction performance on average, but to inspect the individual risk predictions that the model produces. For example, in Chapter 8 we illustrate that some machine learning algorithms can produce biologically implausible models.

2.5.2 Risk classifier

A risk classifier is a model which places patients on an ordinal scale and hence predicts a risk class instead of an event probability. A risk classifier can be derived from any risk prediction model by using threshold values. We do not pursue risk classifiers in this book for reasons stated in Section 2.1.7.

2.5.3 How is prediction modeling different from statistical inference?

A *statistical inference* problem starts by defining the target population and the parameter of interest. Typical parameters are regression coefficients that describe the association of treatment or other exposure with the outcome. Statistical estimates of the parameters are based on a representative sample of the population and a regression model. Goodness-of-fit tests are used to check a model's validity. Confidence intervals are used to express the uncertainty about the estimate of the parameter of interest.

A *statistical prediction* problem also starts by defining a target population, but here the interest is in a personalized parameter because potentially each subject in the population receives a different predicted risk from the model. In other words, a good risk prediction model provides predictions that are useful for each and every individual in the population. Confidence intervals and goodness-of-fit tests are not useful for prediction problems [40]. Application to new patients and cross-validation are used to check a prediction model's validity [32].

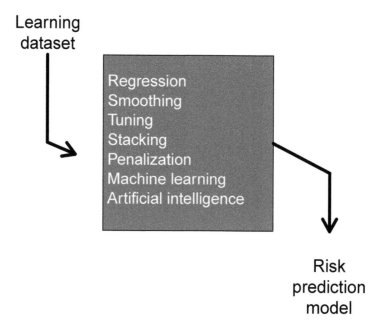

FIGURE 2.5
Illustration of the making of a risk prediction model. A purpose dataset enters on one side, a risk prediction model comes out on the other side. Inside the box, a fully specified modeling algorithm performs all steps of modeling that are needed to fully specify the risk prediction model.

2.5.4 Regression model

Statistical regression models are the basis of many prediction models. They can form the bridge between a database, the observed data (predictors) and unobserved (future) outcomes. Regression models consider much of what we know about the individual patient and put it into a mathematical formula to produce a risk prediction. Logistic and Cox regression models are widely used tools for this task. However, to illustrate the predictive ability of a model resulting from logistic and Cox regression, tables showing odds ratios or hazard ratios are not enough [142, 111]. See also Section 2.7.2. One obvious limitation is that odds ratios and hazard ratios do not have a direct interpretation for the single patient as the predicted risk according to a Cox or logistic regression model depends on the values of the other predictor variables. Additional steps of analysis and ways to present results are needed to describe a prediction model that is based on a regression model. The prediction performance of the model needs to be assessed and compared to benchmark models (Chapters 4 to 6) and presented in a way that facilitates the prediction computations, for example, in the form of a nomogram or Internet risk calculator.

2.5.5 Linear predictor

The linear predictor is a formula which defines how much weight is given to each of the predictor variables. It is used by the classical regression modeling techniques (logistic regression, Cox regression, Fine-Gray regression) and also by penalized regression techniques (LASSO, ridge regression) to formulate a predicted risk for a new patient. For logistic regression, if you know the value of the linear predictor for a new patient, you can then calculate the predicted probability of the event by also using the intercept of the model. For Cox regression models and Fine-Gray regression models, more information is required, such as the baseline hazard function for the Cox model.

2.5.6 Expert selects the candidate predictors

As the person who knows the most about the domain of interest, the expert is in the best position to identify what should be driving the risk of an outcome, regardless of whether the expert has his own experience or literature to support his belief. In many cases the expert could be you or your collaborator. The expert should be interviewed for what he or she feels to be predictive of the outcome of interest, ideally not based on the dataset about to be modeled. We do not want the expert to use, as evidence, many univariable analyses. The message to the modeler is the following: do not pre-analyze the dataset you are bringing to the statistician.

A DAG (directed acyclic graph) is a nice way to get the expert to illustrate how the biology of the system works.

Instead, just think about what should matter, in theory. After identifying that list of variables, it seems best to verify that all of these predictors are routinely available. A prediction model that utilizes a predictor that is only measured in a single institution has drawbacks; dissemination and uptake of the prediction model will be difficult. A base model that relies only upon widely collected predictors has more potential for impact. An enhanced model, featuring a rare predictor, if the predictor variable substantially improves predictive accuracy, is a nice companion model to the base. Next, the domain expert should be queried for direction of effect: for each of the predictors he or she listed, are higher values of the predictor harmful or protective? Asking this question is mostly just a way to remove predictors that the domain expert doesn't really understand. The domain expert ought to have an opinion for each predictor as to direction of effect. Sometimes the domain expert will identify a variable only because a previous study found it to be associated – this is insufficient justification for inclusion in a prediction model.

2.5.7   How to select variables for inclusion in the final model

With all prediction studies, the central question is: which predictor variables should be used? Most importantly, it is generally not sufficient to show significance of a predictor variable in a multiple regression analysis to conclude that the variable is a useful or independent predictor. Indeed, in addition to significance, usually a very large odds ratio or hazard ratio is needed in order to achieve changes of the predicted probabilities that are of a high enough magnitude to trigger a change in the medical or treatment decision or to increase overall prediction accuracy [142, 111].

For example, if the individualized predicted risk of disease changes from 33.1% (conventional predictors alone) to 33.6% (conventional predictors + experimental predictors) then, no matter the true risk, quite likely the value of the two models for medical decision making is equal, at least for this patient profile. A further remark is that the absolute value of odds ratios and hazard ratios are not generally comparable across corresponding predictor variables. It may in some circumstance help to standardize (i.e., to center and scale) the continuous predictors, however, even then the magnitude of the regression coefficients cannot be compared to that of a categorical predictor variable.

Also, the magnitudes of the regression coefficients indicate changes on the linear predictor scale, but these do not directly translate into changes of the absolute risk of the event. This is due to the non-linearity of the model (logit link for logistic regression, cloglog link for Cox regression) and since, the induced change of the predicted absolute risk depends on the baseline risk (the intercept of the linear predictor) and on the other predictor variables.

However, it can be largely unknown in which way the candidate predictors are best combined. Although predictor variables that are correlated with one another do not, per se, cause a problem for making a prediction model, and most machine learning methods have data-adaptive ways to deal with this, highly correlated predictors should typically not be included in the same regression model. A reason for this is that estimating their optimal coefficients via maximum likelihood can be unstable, which can cause computational problems. For constructing the linear predictor, candidate predictors that are near perfectly correlated (collinearity) should not be combined. Transforming continuous variables to have more bell-shaped distributions can improve coefficient estimation stability and thus prediction model performance. These considerations will, in a natural way, lead to a preferably short list of candidate modeling strategies.

2.5.8   All possible interactions

Fishing for all possible interactions is akin to dumping a lot of data into the computer and having it find predictors. Alternatively, the theory-driven approach is argued to produce a more accurate final model. The reason for this is that a human is better at eliminating what might be spurious. The computer is more prone to build a prediction model that relies upon a predictor that will not be predictive in the future. As an example of this, think about a dataset produced by a random number generator. In reality, none of the predictors should work to predict the outcome. By chance, some will appear to predict. A human would not be comfortable with a prediction model based on those predictors; he knows this model cannot last, essentially because the theory behind it is flawed. The computer cannot make this determination so easily.

Having said this, there are times when the theory-driven approach has limitations. For example, one may have a dataset with many potential predictors (e.g., genes) where the theory is not yet mapped out, and these individual predictors may piece together in complex ways. As long as the purpose dataset is restricted to predictors with some plausibility, these large and complex datasets may be best served by machine learning techniques.

2.5.9 Checklist

Checklist modeling strategy

- Describe all steps of modeling from data preparation via variable selection to parameter estimation and formula for prediction.

- Describe all data-dependent steps of modeling such that they can be implemented as computer code, independent of the person who implements them.

- Define the method for dealing with missing values (complete case, multiple imputation, inverse probability weighting, maximum likelihood).

- Define the method for dealing with censored outcome

- Provide the formula or computer code that extracts predictions for outcome at the prediction time horizon from the final model.

2.5.10 Machine learning

A positive side effect of the smartphone epidemic is that artificial intelligence can apply risk prediction models and show results in real time. A smartphone application allows us to use more complex and more appropriate risk prediction models instead of simple and easy-to-memorize ones like the CHA_2DS_2VASC score.[1]

A special form of machine learning, artificial intelligence, continues to learn and train the model when it feels further improvement is possible. This uses an algorithmic approach to modeling instead of the traditional model-based regression approach. Machine learning approaches to prediction were very popular in the early 1990s. They became less popular in the early 2000s but were regaining a lot of popularity in the 2010s with the drastic increase in computer power. Machine learning approaches have some advantages and some disadvantages from a prediction modeling strategy perspective. But first, let us dismiss the hype. Artificial neural networks, based largely on their name, are promoted as being akin to how the human brain works. Even if that were true, that would not necessarily be a good thing given how poor humans tend to be at forming accurate predicted probabilities, especially when humans are compared with traditional statistical approaches [60]. More hype is that machine learning approaches "learn" patterns from the data, because they iterate as they form their weights or structure. Some other statistical methods iterate too, just not so much, and the iteration of the machine learning methods is

---

[1] CHA_2DS_2VASC
C= Congestive heart failure (1 point), H = Hypertension (1 point), A_2 = Age $\geq$ 75 (2 points), D = Diabetes (1 point), S_2 = Stroke (2 points), V = Vascular disease (1 point), A = Age 65-74 (1 point), Sc = Sex category (Female: 1 point)

also what gets them into trouble because too much iteration produces overfit, which predicts poorly (Chapter 8).

2.6 Validation

2.6.1 The conventional model

Fundamentally, the goal of a statistical prediction model is to make the world a better place, i.e., do better than what we can do already. Therefore, the immediate follow-up question for the investigator is, "what model/approach do you currently use for prediction of this outcome?" One of two responses will follow. One, the researcher may respond with "nothing," which should be confirmed by the challenge that "all patients are treated as homogeneous, at uniform risk, and provided with the same risk estimate." Sometimes the follow-up answer is "yes," in which case, the new prediction model just has to be better than the null model. Alternatively, the follow-up answer is "no, clinical judgment is used." In this case, the new model should be compared with clinical judgment. However, if in fact there is an existing statistical model which we could call the *conventional model* (Section 4.4.2), i.e., the answer to the first question was "yes," then we are in a rival model comparison situation (see Chapter 6). The point is, any new model needs to be compared with something else, such as the *conventional model*, clinical judgment, or a rival existing model. If the new model wins the comparison, success has been achieved.

2.6.2 Internal and external validation

Before a prediction model can be applied, it needs to be validated and its expected performance assessed. In machine learning, the expected performance is also called the generalization error [108]. The general parameter for validating a prediction model is prediction performance (Section 2.2).

For this task, validation data are needed. Ideally, these data would be entirely new data collected in a new setting (e.g., new location) for the purpose of calculating accuracy. This is called *external validation*. External validation is most reliable when it is performed by an independent group of researchers. In practice, when external validation data are readily available at the time of model development, they could be merged with the purpose dataset. This is a tradeoff that the modeler must decide. Should the external dataset be left out of the modeling process to be used later for external validation? Or, should these data be merged? Merging the data is the most efficient approach, since more data are used for modeling.

Thus, the best one can do to obtain validation data is to split the available data, such that one part of the data is hidden in the model-building process and then used to calculate accuracy. Unfortunately, splitting the data only once has many disadvantages. The most obvious disadvantage is that the analyst can choose a specific split of the data which produces good-looking results. To avoid this, one has to split the data repeatedly.

> We generally discourage the use of a single split of data into one set for training and one for validation, but see the discussion in Chapter 1. An exception is when the purpose of analysis is only illustration of methods (as in this book).

This process, called cross-validation is the backbone of *internal validation*. Internal cross-validation can be used to tune model parameters (Chapter 8) or assess the predictive performance of a model. The term "internal" can either refer to the fact that the validation study is performed by the same researcher (or team) who made the model, or it can refer to the fact that the validation study (repeatedly) splits the purpose data into training and validation sets (Sections 2.6.5 and 7.4).

2.6.3   Conditional versus expected performance

The following applies to all performance metrics in Section 2.2. This is a subtle point that is often overlooked.

Conditional prediction performance is the performance of a risk prediction model (Figure 2.4) conditional on a single-purpose dataset. A researcher who provides a risk prediction model for clinical application is naturally interested in the conditional performance of the model [59]. The conditional prediction performance can be assessed by an external validation dataset or, with some limitations, using data splitting (Section 7.4).

Expected prediction performance is the performance of a modeling algorithm (Figure 2.5). It is the average performance across all the prediction models that a modeling algorithm can produce using all possible learning datasets of a fixed sample size. A researcher who has invented a new algorithm for building prediction models is naturally interested in the average performance. The expected prediction performance can either be assessed by computer simulation of many datasets or by using cross-validation and bootstrap methods (Section 7.4).

2.6.4   Cross-validation

It is important to understand how well a prediction model is going to do when applied to future patients. Unfortunately, this is never knowable. The best we can do is to simulate the model being applied to future patients. Cross-validation is the way to do this (Section 7.4). With cross-validation we randomly withhold some patients' data to be used as future patients for testing. That is, we pretend we have not seen these patients before and use them for testing a prediction model constructed from the other patients (Section 2.6.5). In its simplest form, cross-validation splits the data into two parts, one time. However, repeated random splitting removes both the investigator and luck.

> *Pretended cross-validation is when variable selection or hyperparameter tuning uses all data and only final fitting is repeated in the loop [Section 7.10.2 in reference 89].*

One must choose the sizes of the training and test sets. Unfortunately, there are only very few general rules for making this decision optimally [166, 163]. In machine learning, 10-fold cross-validation is an established procedure. However, no theory says that 10-fold is always better than 5-fold or 20-fold. Furthermore, it is often necessary to repeat k-fold cross-validation many times in order to have a stable result. Alternatives to k-fold cross-validation are the bootstrap cross-validation and the leave-one-out bootstrap. All these procedures belong under the umbrella term *cross-validation* (Section 7.4).

2.6.5 Data splitting

This simply refers to the act of dividing the purpose dataset into training and test sets (Figure 2.6). To achieve an honest estimate of performance, all data-dependent steps of modeling should be applied in the training data. This includes, for example, data-dependent variable selection. There is no general advice on how much of the data should be used for training or testing (Section 7.4).

Sometimes, in the machine learning literature, a distinction is made between the "validation" and "test" datasets, where with "validation," tuning parameters may be adjusted. Nonetheless, there remains a "test" dataset which represents new data that are applied after no more parameter tuning is done.

2.6.6 Bootstrap

The term bootstrap can refer to many different things in statistics. In the context of this book, bootstrapping is used by certain cross-validation schemes to select subjects for training and validation sets (Section 7.4). Here we distinguish between the re-sampling bootstrap and the sub-sampling bootstrap. With the resampling bootstrap, the training set is obtained by randomly drawing subjects from the purpose dataset *with replacement*. That is, the observation corresponding to a single subject may occur once, several times, or not at all in the learning set. The subjects that do not occur in the bootstrap training set form the bootstrap validation set. The sample size of the bootstrap training set is often chosen to be the same as the sample size of the purpose dataset. It

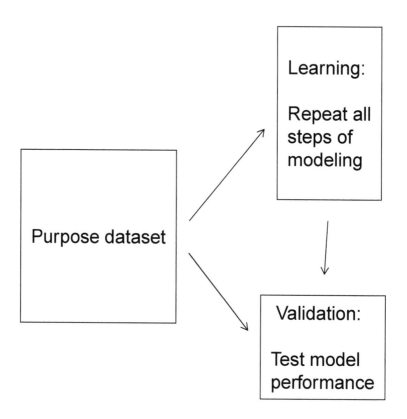

FIGURE 2.6
Internal validation means to split the purpose dataset into non-overlapping training and validation sets.

is possible to leave some subjects out; they are called *out of bag*. Even though some subjects are out of bag, the bootstrap training set can be the same size as the purpose dataset because some subjects appear more than once in the bootstrap training set. With the sub-sampling bootstrap, subjects are also drawn randomly for the bootstrap training set, but *without replacement*. The sub-sampling bootstrap is more robust than the re-sampling bootstrap and thus recommended for high-dimensional problems (more predictor variables than subjects) and complex model-building algorithms [23].

Bootstrapping is also used to construct specific estimators of prediction performance. Bradley Efron has contributed a series of bootstrap estimators that try to correct the optimism of the apparent performance [57, 59]. The apparent performance is obtained by using the full purpose dataset both for model building and to estimate the performance. In this way the performance of the model will be overstated because it is much easier to predict the learning data. A simple "optimism-corrected" bootstrap estimator is obtained by building the model in a bootstrap sample but calculating the performance in the full purpose dataset. In this way one can estimate how much the optimism bias is, and this amount can then be subtracted from the apparent performance to obtain a corrected measure. However, the simple procedure turns out to be inappropriate for data-dependent modeling algorithms; in particular, it does not work well for machine learning methods like random forest (Section 8.3.1), which has near-perfect performance when evaluated in learning data. Efron's .632+ bootstrap is a more sophisticated approach with a broader range of application (Section 7.4).

2.6.7 Model checking and goodness of fit

Classical "model goodness-of-fit tests" are not needed for the purpose of making a prediction model. In fact, they can be misleading, in particular, when the goodness-of-fit statistic is computed in the same dataset which was used to build the model. As the name says, the goodness-of-fit test assesses how well the model fits the current dataset, whereas we are interested in how well the model predicts future patients. Another problem is that usually only one goodness-of-fit aspect of the model can be assessed at a time. For example, consider the aim to include a new continuous predictor variable in a Cox regression model which readily includes demographic variables and a clinical stage. The modeler is concerned, at the same time, with the proportional hazard assumption, the linearity assumption, and the no statistical interaction (effect modification) assumption. While it is not clear in which order the three assumptions should be assessed, the order will potentially affect the resulting model.

The prediction of a regression model usually depends on all aspects and assumptions of a model simultaneously. Thus, instead, model validation with respect to prediction performance is best carried out by comparing the model to a more flexible model which makes fewer assumptions. For example, a standard Cox regression model assumes proportional hazards, linearity of continuous predictor variables, and no interactions between predictor variables. A random survival forest [102] is a flexible model that allows the relaxation of all these assumptions. Thus, if a head-to-head comparison should reveal that the random survival forest has higher prediction accuracy, it means that the standard Cox regression model does not fit very well. Since more flexible models have more parameters, the comparison needs to be well designed and use some form of cross-validation.

See Chapter 5 for details on the accuracy measures. Also, some form of data splitting is needed to make such a comparison fair. See Section 7.4 for more details on cross-validation designs. Chapter 4 describes the regression techniques which rely on a specified model with parametric assumptions and Chapter 8, a bunch of more flexible machine learning methods which can relax these assumptions. When a more flexible model shows more accurate predictions, this indicates that the less flexible model makes too many assumptions.

2.6.8   Reproducibility

It is useful to think of 3 levels of reproducibility. Level 1 is achieved when one statistician provides another with his data and his programming code, and the second statistician obtains the same results as the first. Due to issues like different versions of software and random seeds being different, this does not always happen. Level 2 reproducibility occurs when one statistician provides another with his data and a description of what was done, and the second statistician obtains the same result. The challenge here is with the description being clear and thorough enough to explain to the second statistician all that was done by the first. Due to word limits in journal articles, this level of reproducibility may not always be met. Level 3 reproducibility occurs when one statistician provides another with his data and his results, and the second statistician uses his best judgment to model as he or she prefers, and a near-identical result is achieved. This level of reproducibility is less common.

In the prediction setting this could mean that the predicted risks obtained for the same new patient obtained with one or the other modeling approach, where both approaches are using the same learning dataset, should be so close that the medical implications do not change (e.g., 35.13% risk obtained with a Cox regression model versus 35.29% risk obtained with a random survival forest for the same patient).

2.7 Pitfalls

2.7.1 Age as time scale

In epidemiological cohort studies of exposure-outcome associations it is sometimes useful to use age as the main time scale instead of time-on-study [117, 170]. If age is the time scale, in addition to limitations of follow-up (censored data), the modeler now also has to deal with left truncation (delayed entry). Suppose we set the time origin at age 50 and build a model that predicts the 10-year risk of an event. The patient in our learning dataset for whom follow-up starts at age 58 has eight years delayed entry with respect to the time origin. If this patient had died before age 58, he would not have contributed to the analysis. This is left truncation. A highly readable essay about this type of missing data is given by Hernan [95]. While left truncation can technically be handled by advanced survival analysis [5], the results are usually limited to association parameters such as hazard ratios and cannot easily be transformed into absolute risks. Consider the example where body mass index is one of the predictor variables of a risk prediction model. For a patient who enters with delay, e.g., 8 years after the time origin, the body mass index at the time origin is not available, only the value 8 years after the time origin. In fact, a problem occurs for any predictor variable that changes during life when age is the time scale. Therefore, for the purpose of making a risk prediction model, it is usually very hard to integrate left truncation in a modeling framework that uses age as the time scale.

Let us explain the obstacles further by considering the prediction model framework of Section 2.1, now with age as main time scale. First, we set the time origin. For the sake of our example, this is age 50. Hence, the model can only be applied to subjects exactly at age 50. We need to vary the time origin across the age scale and work with multiple time origins in order to obtain risk predictions at other ages. The next problem is due to the fact that, typically, the predictor variables are only measured at a single age for each subject. For any fixed time origin, say age 50, the risk prediction of a new subject can be based on those subjects in the purpose dataset who were alive and event-free at age 50. But, for how many subjects in the purpose dataset who are alive and event-free at age 50, do we actually have measurements of the predictor variables taken exactly at age 50? In order to make a meaningful risk prediction model, it is necessary that either (1) all predictor variables are constant across age or (2) repeated longitudinal measurements of the age-dependent predictor variables are available. For example, consider that body mass index (BMI) is one of the predictor variables. A subject who enters the study at age 41 and stays alive and event-free until age 50 can contribute to a prediction of the risk at time origin age 50. However, if the BMI of this subject was only measured at age 41, it may have increased or decreased considerably in the following 9 years.

2.7.2 Odds ratios and hazard ratios are not predictions of risks

Many applied researchers conclude that a new biomarker or other predictor variable is *predictive* or an *independent predictor* simply because it shows a significant odds ratio in a multiple logistic regression analysis or a significant hazard ratio in a multiple Cox regression analysis. However, this is often not justified for many different reasons [116, 142]. A general problem with this interpretation is that odds ratios and hazard ratios alone are not sufficient to predict what the patient is interested in [110], that is, a personalized probability of survival chances (or of the risk of an event). In addition to the odds ratios (hazard ratios) of all predictor variables, the personalized predicted risk depends on the predictor values of the patient and the intercept in logistic regression and the baseline hazard function in Cox regression.

Let us illustrate the situation by means of a real example. The study by Henke et al. [94] randomized head and neck cancer patients to epo or placebo for the control of their anemia. The results of the trial showed a very large odds ratio (OR) for epo treatment: OR= 90.92 $CI_{95} : [23.9; 493.4], p < 0.0001$ in a multivariable Cox regression model which was adjusted for age, gender, baseline hemoglobin value, resection status (complete, incomplete, no surgery possible). This extremely high odds ratio might lead the reader to conclude that all patients should receive the treatment. However, for many patients the anemia will resolve by itself, i.e., on the placebo treatment. If an individual patient already has a chance of resolution of anemia without treatment, the attractiveness of epo treatment shrinks substantially. For example, based on the logistic regression model, the predicted probability that a 51-year-old man with complete tumor resection and baseline hemoglobin level 12.6 *g/dl* reaches the target hemoglobin level is 97.4% with epo treatment and 29.2% under placebo treatment. For this patient the expected treatment effect is large. If an otherwise similar patient has baseline hemoglobin level 14.8 *g/dl*, then the same logistic regression model predicts a 99.8% chance of treatment success with epo treatment and 84.7% under placebo. For this patient the expected treatment effect is not as large. Therefore, although the odds ratio of 90.92 applies to both patients, the first patient is far more likely to choose treatment while the second patient is likely to let the anemia go away on its own. In conclusion, this example shows that the odds ratio of one factor (here: treatment) is not sufficient to provide personalized prediction.

2.7.3 Do not blame the metric

It is disappointing for a researcher to find that his/her new biomarker does not increase prediction performance. This is particularly true when the new biomarker showed significance in a multivariable logistic regression model or Cox regression model. One reason can be that the effect of the biomarker, though significant, is of too small magnitude [116, 142]. In search for an alternative explanation in this situation, some researchers have accused the performance metrics of being insensitive [140]. While this has led to the invention of overly sensitive metrics [98, 141], it seems that what is really needed is a better understanding of the difference between a regression coefficient and the prediction performance metrics. The regression coefficients (e.g., as odds ratios or hazard ratios) have a conditional interpretation given the other predictor variables in the model, and they do not depend on the distribution of the biomarker in the population. The prediction performance metrics are unconditional population parameters that depend on the distribution of the biomarker in the population, as we illustrate in the following.

Let us consider a hypothetical (computer-simulated) situation where a binary biomarker (negative/positive) has a hazard ratio of 2.5 under a Cox-Weibull regression model. The estimate and interpretation of the hazard ratio in a multivariable Cox regression model does not depend on *how many subjects* in the target population have a positive biomarker value. However, the prediction performance of the Cox regression model does depend on the (marginal) distribution of the biomarker. Figure 2.7 illustrates this based on simulated data with a survival outcome. We set the prediction time horizon at 5 years and simulate two predictor variables: a continuous predictor variable with normal distribution, which represents the only variable in a conventional Cox regression model, and a binary variable that represents the new biomarker added to the conventional Cox regression model. The probability of a positive biomarker value in the simulated population is varied from very low to very high. Two independent datasets are simulated for training and validation, both with sample size n = 20,000. The training dataset is used to fit the conventional Cox regression model and the experimental Cox regression model which adds the new biomarker. The validation data are used to calculate the 5-year AUC and the 5-year IPA (see Chapter 5). Figure 2.7 shows that even with very large samples, the (increase of the) prediction performance by the new biomarker will be low if very few or very many subjects in the target population are biomarker positive.

Thus, in the case of a low biomarker frequency, insensitivity is not the fault of the metric but can be explained by the fact that few subjects of the target population have a beneficial effect from adding the biomarker. Consequently, a significant hazard ratio with a high magnitude but insignificant increase of prediction performance may mean that there is a subgroup of the target population where the prediction performance is increased significantly but this subgroup is too small to change the performance in the total target population. In summary, to achieve a high increase in the IPA and AUC by a binary marker, one needs all of the following:

- a reasonably large hazard ratio of the marker in a multivariable model,

- that the marker is not too correlated with the other predictor variables,

- that the fraction of marker positive subjects is not too small (or too large).

Similar considerations can be made for continuous markers where a reasonably large spread (standard deviation) is needed to achieve a high increase in the IPA and AUC.

2.7.4   Censored data versus competing risks

It is useful to stringently distinguish between the biological system which describes what happens to the subjects/patients (over time) from the observational pattern which limits the available information about when and what will happen to the subjects in their (individual) follow-up periods.

> *Treating competing risks as censoring may lead to an analysis of life after death.*

The term *competing risk* typically refers to a new biological state which typically changes the risk of the event of interest. For example, when the competing risk is death, then after death the risk of the event of interest changes from any positive value to zero. An example of a non-fatal competing risk occurs in a patient who is diagnosed with primary biliary cirrhosis (PBC) in the liver when he receives a liver transplant. Then, after the patient has received the transplant, the risks of death and other PBC-related events change.

The term *censoring* typically refers to the limitations that the data analyst may have regarding the knowledge of the biological states of some subjects in parts of the observation period. The most extreme form of *censoring* is when the information about a subject is completely missing, all the way from the time origin to the prediction time horizon.

> *Censoring is like a black stripe which hides words or parts of a sentence of a* ▮▮▮▮▮▮ *article.*

There are two pitfalls related to the confusion of *censoring* and *competing risks*. The first pitfall occurs when competing risks are unintentionally treated as censored, for example, when using the methods Kaplan-Meier and Cox regression to predict the absolute risk of an event when there are competing risks [81, 157]. This would often lead to a hypothetical world in which the competing risks cannot occur, and in the extreme case one could erroneously study the quality of life after death. This happens because the Kaplan-Meier and Cox regression methods assume that a censored observation would later experience the event.

The other pitfall occurs when the reason for the end of follow-up (censored) depends on the current medical state of the patient and is not predictable based on the information available at baseline. Many statistical procedures will lead to biased results if the length of the follow-up depends on the rate of the event of interest.

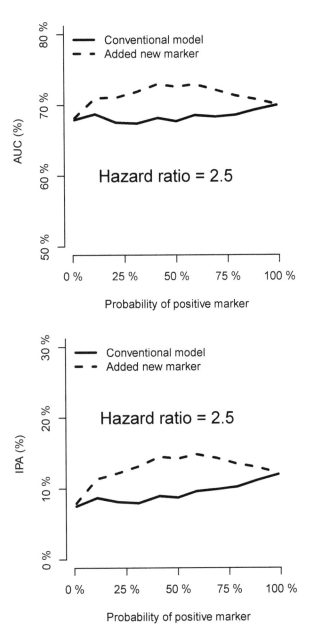

FIGURE 2.7
Rare biomarkers do not have much predictive power. Shown are results based on simulated data where the hazard ratio of the biomarker has the value 2.5 regardless of the prevalence of the marker. The effects of the biomarker on the discrimination ability (AUC), shown in the upper panel, and on the overall predictive performance (IPA), shown in the lower panel, are diminishing when the prevalence of the biomarker is either extremely low or extremely high.

2.7.5 Disease-specific survival

Disease-specific survival is a popular outcome in cancer research when there are competing risks. However, it should be avoided in particular when the aim is prediction. The reason is that disease-specific survival does not have a clinically meaningful interpretation for the patient. It is the probability of not dying of the disease of interest assuming another cause of death does not occur, which is hypothetical. Instead one should treat death due to other causes as competing risks and predict the absolute risk of disease-specific death (cumulative incidence).

2.7.6 Overfitting

Overfitting is a serious threat to each prediction model. Overfitting means that the model is better at predicting the individuals in the dataset that were used for making the model than it is at predicting the individuals in the background population or future patients. A more complex model will often outperform a less complex model in the training data. One drawback to the complex model is that it is often unclear if the more complex model predicts yet unseen patients more accurately. And since more complex models often issue more extreme predictions that could motivate subjects to make a decision, it is important to not only compare the average performance but also look into outliers in the personalized predictions when comparing a complex model to a simple model.

Overfitting has many faces. A generic example is the following. We try to learn from a dataset about the predictor-outcome relationship in the target population, but we learn things that are specific to the subjects in the learning dataset and do not generalize to the target population.

One should note that near-perfect prediction performance is suspicious in most applications, and one should check the data, the algorithm and the corresponding computer code for flaws when the value of the prediction performance metric takes an extreme value.

2.7.7 Data-dependent decisions

While all prediction models need to be validated, for the purpose of developing a useful prediction model it is particularly essential that all the data-dependent steps are applied in each learning set during cross-validation. If, for example, variables are selected by a manual or automated forward or backward model selection procedure, then the stability of the resulting model should be validated. This can be done by using a cross-validation procedure where the entire selection process is repeated in subsets or sub-samples of the data (Section 7.4). Such a validation may reveal that results are notoriously unstable. See [14] for an example.

2.7.8 Balancing data

In machine learning, some algorithms "tremble when faced with imbalanced classification data" [4]. When the aim is to make a risk prediction model for medical research, the data are never balanced, i.e., it is very unlikely that the overall probability of the event of interest within the prediction time horizon is exactly 50%. Sometimes model developers will construct purpose datasets that are balanced with respect to outcome using oversampling, undersampling or synthetic data generation. While this might maximize statistical power, that is not the goal in a prediction modeling context. It may also be believed that this balance will produce a more accurate prediction model than one based on data that has the outcome frequency occurring naturally. The problem is that, although balancing the data with respect to outcome may help the model to maximize its discriminative ability (AUC), the model will be miscalibrated when applied to future cases, because when applied again, the model will not encounter data that are balanced in the same way. The predicted probabilities will be incorrect unless further correction is made.

2.7.9 Independent predictor

A common procedure is to first run univariate analyses, where each of the candidate experimental predictors is tested by itself for association with outcome. Then, the "significant" experimental predictors are assessed in a multiple regression model where they are combined with the conventional predictors into a new regression model. Here either (1) each of the significant experimental predictors is tested by itself together with conventional predictors or (2) all of the significant experimental predictors are tested as a group in combination with the conventional predictors. In fact, this ad hoc strategy is a special case of a stepwise forward selection algorithm (Section 2.7.10). Commonly it is then concluded that the experimental predictors that remain significant in multiple regression analyses are "independent predictors." However, different additional analytical methods that target the prediction performance need to be applied in order to draw conclusions of this type. We refer to Section 6.4 where the aim is to analyze if a new predictor variable adds information to an existing risk prediction model.

2.7.10 Automated variable selection

It should be noted that most forms of stepwise regression, with backward elimination being the most prominent variant, despite being very popular, cannot be recommended when applied naively [67, 14]. This is particularly so when the purpose is to build a risk prediction model where some form of cross-validation is required to achieve generalizability to new patients. Frank Harrell [87] has some important remarks about stepwise variable selection (forward and backward): effect sizes are exaggerated, p-values are systematically too small, confidence intervals too narrow, and most devastatingly, it allows the analyst not to think.

3

How should I prepare for modeling?

A statistical risk prediction model is a formula that weights predictors and calculates personalized risks. The weights depend on parameters that have to be estimated from data. The model learns the relationship between the predictors and the outcome from what happened to previous patients. To prepare for modeling, a dataset has to be constructed which contains predictor variables and event time outcomes from previous patients. This chapter discusses the many data preparation issues (see Figure 3.1) associated with the overall goal, which is to develop a risk prediction model for implementation in clinical, public health, or other real-life settings. In most applied statistical projects, the majority of the time is spent on preparation of the data, not on the actual statistical analysis. It is therefore critical that the modeler thinks through all of the issues discussed in this chapter before any statistical data analysis is conducted.

3.1 Definition of subjects

Risk predictions are only useful and applicable when targeted at a specific group of patients. Ideally, the data used to build the model are representative of this group, for example, a random sample. Often the patients whose data are included in the database satisfied certain inclusion and exclusion criteria in a certain calendar period. Sometimes the data were originally collected for a different purpose, e.g., a cohort study or a randomized clinical trial. No matter how the data were obtained, in order to know if a prediction model can be used on a new patient, it is necessary to know (the limitations of) the dataset behind the model.

We illustrate some of the steps that are needed in order to construct a purpose dataset by referring to a popular risk prediction tool: the NIH Risk Assessment Tool.[1] The disclaimer of the NIH risk calculator states that the risk prediction is based on an equation (i.e., a model) that was derived in the Framingham study data. It seems that the tool is applicable to all patients. However, this is not quite true. For example, a person aged 80 or older and

---

[1]http://cvdrisk.nhlbi.nih.gov/

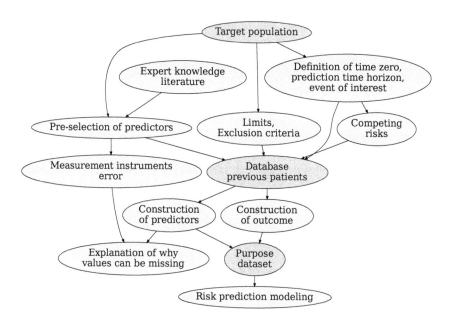

FIGURE 3.1
Steps in moving from a database which contains data from previous patients to constructing the purpose dataset which is the basis of risk prediction modeling.

a person aged 40 or younger or cannot get a prediction from this tool. The reason is the following: when the tool is applied to a new person's predictor variables, the dataset is searched for persons with similar characteristics. The prediction is an appropriate summary of what happened to the persons in the dataset within a 10-year period. Thus, if the dataset behind the model equation included no persons outside the age range 40 to 79 then there are no persons similar to a person aged younger than 40 or older than 79 and hence the tool cannot be applied without extrapolating into the no-evidence-based region.

At this point, one should also note that the uncertainty of the predictions issued by a tool would generally be expected to be relatively low for persons who are similar to many profiles in the dataset and relatively high for persons whose profile occurs rarely in the dataset. For example, one would expect that a 50-year-old would get a more reliable prediction as compared to a 79-year-old person when the dataset included more persons around 50 than persons around 79 years. Generally, when more predictors are added to the purpose dataset (to be included in the modeling process) the problem of outliers in the covariate space becomes more severe.

It seems to be a real problem when a risk calculator can be applied to a rare combination of covariate values or even to a biologically impossible combination of covariate values. To explain this problem in a less abstract way, consider the statement of a nomogram [114]. The result from the risk calculation starts the message for the patient by saying "Mr. X, if we had 100 men exactly like you, ..." The patient should ask back "Doc, how many patients exactly like me have you seen?"

3.2 Choice of time scale

In Section 2.1 we described the need to set a time origin which is typically a diagnosis, treatment, or sometimes the beginning of being under surveillance.

No matter exactly how a predictor variable is measured or derived, it is most important that only information from before or up to the time origin is used. An unfortunate violation of this principle is sometimes termed *conditioning on the future* [8]. This would result in a non-applicable model because a model which depends on values that are first realized after the time origin cannot produce a risk prediction for the new patient when the prediction is needed. Technically speaking, we should mention that it is allowed that the modeling algorithm makes use of all values of the previous patients, but input to the risk prediction model must not depend on future values of a predictor variable.

The NIH Risk Assessment Tool predicts a person's risk of suffering a heart attack in the next 10 years. Thus, in this example, the predicted event is *heart attack* and the prediction horizon is *10 years*. It is not said what time zero should be. A reasonable interpretation of the 10-year risk seems to be that this is the risk in the period between now and 10 years from now. Also, this means that the cholesterol and blood pressure measurements, as well as the smoking status, are to be evaluated. In association studies, some modelers would prefer age, rather than time on study, as the time scale. When the aim is to make a risk prediction model, using age as the time scale is not advised because the only age zero that all subjects have in common is birth (see also Section 2.7.1). But, rarely are all subjects that contribute to the purpose dataset followed from birth. More commonly the predictor variables are time-varying but measured only once at a certain age for each subject in the purpose dataset. So, when age is the time scale, it is possible to make a risk prediction model that can be used at any age (as time zero) and a user of the model can update the personalized predicted risk every year using updated values of the time-varying predictor variables. But, such a model requires a purpose dataset that is rich enough to represent the target population at any of the many possible time origins (ages).

3.3   Pre-selection of predictor variables

Our philosophy is that the subject matter expert should initially select the predictor variables to be included in the model [139]. A benefit of having the domain expert identify the predictors is enhanced physician buy-in, in that users are more likely to have faith in the model when it includes all the predictors that they think should be present. If a physician thinks that either the prediction model lacks a very important predictor or the prediction model contains a predictor that is nonsense yet influential, the physician is unlikely to use this prediction model. A prediction model that is not used at all is not very helpful to anybody. The choice of predictors should then be confirmed by a systematic review of the literature.

A good way to communicate the selection of predictors is a box-arrow diagram or DAG (directed acyclic graph). An example is shown in Figure 3.2. Such a graph indicates which variables are believed to affect the risk of the event of interest and how (directly or indirectly). A DAG is both useful in the preparation of the modeling, and also at a later stage to check the plausibility of results. Further, such a diagram can help to reveal redundant variables as well to identify unobserved predictors (see Figure 3.2). It may also indicate which variables are believed to mediate or modify the effect of other predictors.

We need to choose candidate predictors from the list of available predictors. Available predictors are those that have non-missing values for the majority

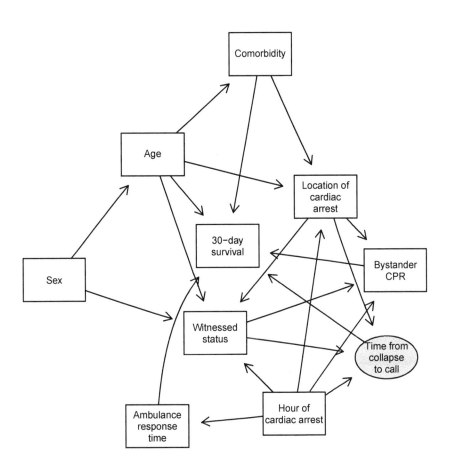

FIGURE 3.2
Example of a DAG, which indicates how predictors of cardiac arrest patients are believed to affect 30-day survival. The variables *hour and location of arrest* and *witnessed status* are not believed to have a direct influence on the outcome. The *time from collapse to call of an ambulance* is not known to the analyst but believed to be an important predictor of 30-day survival.

of the patients in the purpose dataset and are also affordable and accessible in due course when the prediction model is to be used on a future patient.

Candidate predictors include all variables that are believed to be associated with substantial changes of the event risk. Importantly, by "believed" we mean external knowledge and not results derived from the purpose dataset. Also, by "substantial" we mean a change of predicted risk which is meaningful for the patient. The decision regarding which variables should serve as predictors should be made prior to the examination of relationships in the purpose dataset to be modeled. For the believed predictors it should further be possible to note in which direction changes of the predictor variable will affect the predicted risk. For example, in many cases increasing age will imply increasing risk. Again, this is an external expert pre-knowledge which should be obtained without using the data.

In addition to the believed predictors, the candidate predictors include experimental variables. These are variables that are of specific interest for the current research study but their predictive performance has not been studied.

A final recommendation is that, in competing risk settings, one should use variables that affect the competing risk even if they do not directly affect the event of interest. Such variables will help identify subjects at high or low risk of the competing risk. A subject with a high risk of the competing risk is naturally at (relatively) lower risk of the event of interest. Hence, even if the variable is not biologically related to the risk of the event of interest it may indirectly help to improve the risk prediction model.

3.4 Preparation of predictor variables

For each predictor variable considered, as well as for the outcome, a protocol should detail the way measurements are taken and perhaps mention measurement or detection bias. Such a protocol can be called a "data dictionary"; see Table 3.1 for an example. If indicated, one could also list acceptable alternative ways to obtain measurement.

A predictor variable can be categorical (i.e., discrete), ordinal (categorical with a logical ordering of the categories), or continuous. For each of these variable types, we now discuss how to include them in the purpose dataset (Sections 3.4.1 and 3.4.2).

There are several useful ways to further characterize predictor variables. One way is the expense of collection either in monetary or inconvenience terms (pain or time). Another is conventional versus experimental. Conventional variables are expected to be present in the model. Experimental predictors are thought to potentially add predictive value but have not been thoroughly evaluated. Time-varying predictor variables need special attention. If a marker is measured repeatedly for all patients, then any parameter of the time-series

TABLE 3.1

Example of a data dictionary. Column `Name` is the name of the variable in the purpose dataset; `Label` is text as it should appear in research output; `Unit/Levels` are the measurement units (continuous variables) and levels (categorical variables) as they appear in the purpose dataset and in the research output; and `Expected effect` is the known (conventional predictors) or hypothesized (experimental predictors) effects on the risk of the event of interest.

Name	Label	Unit/Levels	Expected effect
age	Age at entry	Years	positive
gend	Sex	1=Female	lower risk
		2=Male	higher risk
spouse	Living with spouse	Yes	lower risk
	No spouse/living alone	No	higher risk
...	...	...	...
pckyrs	Smoking history	packyears	positive
sbp	Systolic blood pressure	mmHg	positive

up to the time origin can be a new derived predictor variable (Sections 3.4.3 and 3.4.4).

3.4.1 Categorical variables

For all categorical variables, one should record the possible categories and, when necessary, an additional explanation. For example, a variable called "sex" could have possible categories "0" and "1" where the additional explanation is that "0" means "female" and "1" means "male." A categorical variable which can take on many values may need to be adapted to the sample size and number of events. For example, the potential range of values of the Charlson comorbidity index can be 0 to 37 [130]. However, when for example only a few patients in the purpose dataset had a Charlson comorbidity score above 3, then it can be necessary to collapse this variable into fewer categories and for example, define three levels: $0, 1 - 2, \geq 3$. These modifications can all be performed using basic commands in most statistical software packages.

3.4.2 Continuous variables

For all continuous variables, one should record the lowest and highest possible values and, if available, normal population reference values. This is in order to define sanity checks and to detect outliers. In addition to the units of measurement it is always useful to provide additional information regarding the measurement device and the measurement method. For example, there are many different ways to measure blood pressure, so it is useful to provide a certain level of clarity regarding how the measure is taken. This detail can also add clinical nuance that is not available in any other way.

3.4.3 Derived predictor variables

A predictor variable can be derived from one or several of the other variables in the database. For predictor variables that are derived from other variables, we need the explicit formula or computer algorithm that calculates their value for the new patients. A simple example of a derived predictor variable is body mass index (BMI) categorized as (normal, overweight, obese). The BMI is calculated on a continuous scale from body weight and body height measurements using the well-known formula and then categorized using population reference values. For illustration consider the following sample:

```
# R-code
library(Publish)
data(Diabetes)
Diabetes[1:5,c("weight","height")]
```

id	weight	height
1	121	62
2	218	64
3	256	61
4	119	67
5	183	68

The following R-code first transforms from pound lb/in to kg/m and then defines the common BMI categories.

```
# R-code
Diabetes$height.m <-  Diabetes$height*0.0254
Diabetes$weight.kg <-  Diabetes$weight*0.4535929
Diabetes$bmi <-  Diabetes$weight.kg/Diabetes$height.m^2
Diabetes$BMI <- cut(Diabetes$bmi,c(0,18,25,30,Inf),labels=c("
    UnderWeight","NormalWeight","OverWeight","Obese"))
Diabetes[,c("weight","height","bmi","BMI")]
```

id	weight	height	bmi	BMI
1	121	62	22.13099	NormalWeight
2	218	64	37.41927	Obese
3	256	61	48.37034	Obese
4	119	67	18.63787	NormalWeight
5	183	68	27.82480	OverWeight

Another example of a derived predictor variable is renal impairment which enters the EUROSCORE http://www.euroscore.org/calc.html as a function of patient's age, gender, body weight and plasma creatinine. At this point, we should note that it rarely makes sense to include a derived variable and also one or more of its ingredients into a model. It then depends on the nature of the modeling algorithm and the sample size of the purpose dataset whether one should use the derived variable or its ingredients. One should also be aware of the fact that complex derived variables such as a Charlson comorbidity score will often have slightly varying definition and frequently cannot be directly compared between studies. In the preparation of the statistical modeling one should, therefore, be very specific regarding how exactly the derived variables are obtained and ideally provide the software code.

3.4.4 Repeated measurements

For variables that change over time (time-varying variables) it may make sense to include repeated measurements from the same patient as predictors. A simple example is the so-called "last value carried forward" which, for each patient, is the measurement of the variable which is closest in time to the time origin and still measured earlier than the time origin. This may or may not make sense depending on the situation and one should consider the time-frequency of measurements within the patient and the homogeneity of the measurement time-pattern across patients.

More complex examples of predictor variables that are derived from repeated measurements occur in prostate cancer studies. Here repeated measurements of the prostate-specific antigen (PSA) are routinely summarized into single values per patient. For example, the PSA doubling time is derived from a linear regression model fitted to the log-transformed measurements of the last one or two years before the time origin. For illustration purposes, consider the data shown in Table 3.2 and Figure 3.3 which contains the longitudinal PSA measurements of two subjects.

The following R-code first computes the number of days since the first measurements, then restricts to the first 2 years, and finally computes the PSA doubling time based on a linear model fitted to the PSA values on the logarithmic scale (3.3).

```
# R-code
library(data.table)
setDT(long)
long <- long[,list("psa.time"=psadate-psadate[1],psadate,psa),by=
    subject]
long <- long[psa.time<=(2*365.25),]
# psa doubling time formula
psadt <- function(time,value){ # input date and psa value
    (log(2)/coef(lm(log(value)~time))[2])/365.25 # lm is linear model
}
# now apply function to individual subjects
```

TABLE 3.2
Longitudinal measurements of prostate-specific antigen (psa) for two subjects.

subject	psadate	psa
1	1996-05-20	5.1
1	1996-08-12	8.1
1	1996-11-04	11.0
1	1997-01-27	12.8
1	1997-04-28	18.9
1	1997-07-21	24.2
1	1997-10-13	46.3
1	1998-01-05	65.2
1	1998-03-23	131.0
2	1996-07-04	97.8
2	1996-10-03	62.0
2	1997-01-02	69.5
2	1997-04-08	72.9
2	1997-06-12	72.6
2	1997-08-28	73.4
2	1997-11-20	80.6
2	1998-02-12	84.8
2	1998-05-05	93.3

```
long[,list("psa.doublingtime"=psadt(psa.time,psa)),by=subject]
```

TABLE 3.3
PSA doubling times computed based on the data shown in Table 3.2.

subject	psa.doublingtime
1	0.42
2	9.39

3.4.5 Measurement error

Predictor variables that are difficult to measure are to be used with great care. When randomness in the value of a predictor variable translates into randomness of the predicted risk, it may happen that a patient bases an important decision about the medical future on information which, to a great extent, is subject to randomness. Hence, measurement error in one or more predictor variables can be a serious problem for a risk prediction model. A general goal is to reduce measurement error for all predictors to as low as possible. While this is often not under the control of the modeler, the data dictionary (Table

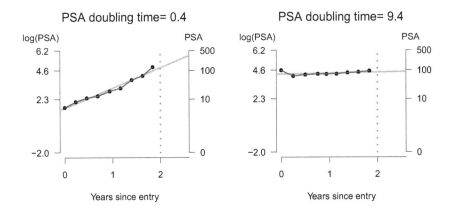

FIGURE 3.3
Longitudinal prostate-specific antigen (PSA) measurements of two patients
collected in a two-year period after the start of an active surveillance program.
The solid gray lines show the best linear approximations of the PSA time-
process after logarithmic transformation.

3.1) should clearly define how each predictor was measured. For example, the
NIH Risk Assessment Tool uses the systolic blood pressure and the web link
explains: Systolic blood pressure is the first number of your blood pressure
reading. For example, if your reading is 120/80 (120 over 80), your systolic
blood pressure is 120. The page does not explain further circumstances of
measurement such as the time of the day, number of repetitions, position of
body, or if a medically trained person should perform the measurement. These
circumstances, as well as the age of the last blood pressure measurement at
the time origin, may affect the value of the blood pressure reading and hence
the predicted risk.

3.4.6   Missing values

When values of a variable are missing in the database, one should try hard
to find the possible reasons for the missingness. For example, a value can be
missing because it was not entered correctly into the computer, or because
the patient did not show up at the examination, or the patient was in too bad
of condition to perform the measurement on that day. The documentation of
the reasons for the missingness is important because most statistical modeling
strategies rely on untestable assumptions regarding the mechanism, which
decide why a measurement is available for one patient and not for another

patient. It is generally not useful to separate the process of data imputation from the process of modeling (Section 7.5).

3.5   Preparation of event time outcome

At this point, it should be clear which event the risk prediction model should predict and at what time point the prediction should be given to the patient (see Section 2.1). The first step is to define which subjects of the database are eligible for the purpose dataset with respect to the time origin. One can only include subjects in the purpose dataset who are alive at the time origin and for whom the event of interest did not occur before the time origin. The second step is to compute the time between the date of the time origin and the end of follow-up. For each subject, the end of follow-up is the earliest of the date of

code 1 the event of interest

code 2 a competing risk (such as death without event)

code 0 last contact (lost to follow-up, censored).

Refer to Sections 2.4.5 and 2.4.6 and 2.7.4 for more explanations of the terms *censored* and *competing risks*. In the following we explain how to prepare the outcome information in the purpose dataset in the form of **two variables**, the *time variable* and the *event variable*. The *time variable* is the difference between the subject-specific date of the end of follow-up and the subject-specific date of the time origin. It is a numeric variable with time units such as days, months or years since the time origin. The *event variable* takes on coded values, 1 for the event of interest, 2 for the competing risks (if any), 0 for censored. In situations with multiple competing risks, one can either use codes 3, 4, etc., or code all competing risks with value 2. The latter is the most common; the former makes sense when the modeling algorithm needs to differentiate between the different competing risks (e.g., the risk factor influences differ across the competing risks).

3.5.1   Illustration without competing risks

Consider a setting which resembles the one of the CHA_2DS_2VASC prediction score [71]. Patients are included when they are diagnosed with atrial fibrillation. The date of diagnosis with atrial fibrillation is the time origin (`af.date`). Suppose first that the event of interest is all-cause death. In a cohort study, patients are followed until date of death (`death.date`) or 1st of January 2015, whatever comes first. Here are data from 5 hypothetical patients:

id	af.date	death.date	lost.date
1	2001-04-25	–	–
2	1995-02-16	2011-10-27	–
3	2001-09-09	–	–
4	1999-12-20	2009-01-02	–
5	1997-05-27	–	2008-08-17

To calculate the event time outcome using these data, we apply the following R-code.

```
# R-code (no competing risks)
d$af.date <- as.Date(d$af.date)
d$death.date <- as.Date(d$death.date)
d$lost.date <- as.Date(d$lost.date)
d$time <- pmin(  # parallel minimum
    d$death.date, # event
    d$lost.date,  # lost to follow-up
    as.Date("2015-01-01") # administrative censoring
    ,na.rm=TRUE)-d$af.date # date of subject specific time origin
d$event <- 0 # initialize all subjects
d[!is.na(d$death.date),]$event <- 1 # event
d
```

id	af.date	death.date	lost.date	time	event
1	2001-04-25	NA	NA	4999 days	0
2	1995-02-16	2011-10-27	NA	6097 days	1
3	2001-09-09	NA	NA	4862 days	0
4	1999-12-20	2009-01-02	NA	3301 days	1
5	1997-05-27	NA	2008-08-17	4100 days	0

3.5.2 Illustration with competing risks

Now suppose that *stroke* is the event of interest and *death without stroke* is a competing risk. The data of the five hypothetical patients (Section 3.5.1) are now enhanced with one more variable: the date of stroke:

id	af.date	death.date	stroke.date	lost.date
1	2001-04-25	–	2005-11-16	–
2	1995-02-16	2011-10-27	–	–
3	2001-09-09	–	–	–
4	1999-12-20	2009-01-02	2007-09-01	–
5	1997-05-27	–	1999-12-18	2008-08-17

To calculate the event time variable with competing risks using these data, we apply the following R-code.

```
# R-code (with competing risks)
d$af.date <- as.Date(d$af.date)
```

```
d$stroke.date <- as.Date(d$stroke.date)
d$death.date <- as.Date(d$death.date)
d$lost.date <- as.Date(d$lost.date)
d$time <- pmin(  # parallel minimum
  d$stroke.date, # event
  d$death.date,  # competing risk
  d$lost.date,   # lost to follow-up
  as.Date("2015-01-01") # administrative censoring
  ,na.rm=TRUE) -d$af.date # date of subject specific time origin
d$event <- 0 # initialize all subjects
d[!is.na(d$stroke.date),]$event <- 1
d[!is.na(d$death.date) & is.na(d$stroke.date),]$event <- 2
d
```

id	af.date	death.date	stroke.date	lost.date	event	time
1	2001-04-25	NA	2005-11-16	NA	1	1666 days
2	1995-02-16	2011-10-27	NA	NA	2	6097 days
3	2001-09-09	NA	NA	NA	0	4862 days
4	1999-12-20	2009-01-02	2007-09-01	NA	1	2812 days
5	1997-05-27	NA	1999-12-18	2008-08-17	1	935 days

3.5.3   Artificial censoring at the prediction time horizon

In some situations, it is useful to censor all events and the competing risk(s) that occur **after** the prediction time horizon. The argument for doing this could be that the model should not learn about the risk of the event within the prediction time horizon from events that occur after the prediction time horizon. Whether such artificial censoring is useful depends on the specific modeling algorithm. In fact, it can be considered as part of the modeling algorithm. The idea is straightforward to implement with or without competing risks. The time variable is truncated at the time horizon and for subjects who experience an event or a competing risk **after** the date of the prediction time horizon, so we set the event variable to value 0 (zero is the code for right-censored in most software packages).

For the purpose of illustration, consider the data prepared at the end of Section 3.5.2 and set the prediction time horizon at 5 years. We truncate the time variable at 5 years and set the corresponding event variable to the code value 0.

```
# R-code
d$time.5 <- pmin(d$time,5*365.25)
d$event.5 <- d$event
d[d$time>5*365.25,]$event.5 <- 0
d[,c("time","event","time.5","event.5")]
```

time	event	time.5	event.5
1666 days	1	1666.00 days	1
6097 days	2	1826.25 days	0
4862 days	0	1826.25 days	0
2812 days	1	1826.25 days	0
935 days	1	935.00 days	1

As can be seen in the table, all event-free follow-up time and all events that occur after the prediction time horizon (1826.25 days) have been removed from the purpose dataset.

4

I am ready to build a prediction model

At this point, you now have a purpose dataset in your hands. We will walk you through what you need to do with it in order to produce a formula that predicts risks in future patients. The general approach to model building depends on the type and observational pattern of the outcome (Section 4.1). For each outcome, we show how to obtain a *benchmark model* for prediction (Section 4.2) and introduce our concept of the *conventional model*. The benchmark and conventional models will play a central role in the interpretation of prediction performance discussed in Chapters 5 and 6. We then go on to explain how to include predictor variables and how to obtain risk predictions from standard regression models (Section 4.3). We address the three different settings that correspond to the three outcome types: uncensored binary, right-censored without competing risks, and right-censored with competing risks. Throughout, we illustrate these methods using the data of the *in vitro fertilization study*, the *oral cancer study* and the *prostate cancer active surveillance study*.

The final task is to spell out a modeling strategy for the current dataset and research aim. As in chess, it is better to have a bad strategy than no strategy. However, it is challenging to provide an overall modeling strategy for a couple of reasons. One, there is not a single strategy that is universally agreed upon to be optimal. Two, there is little data to support one modeling strategy over another. As a result, we will provide our approach that we tend to use, and we will do our best to explain why we do things this way (Section 4.4). While we have many years of experience, we are hard-pressed to claim this strategy is the optimal one in all instances. In this chapter, we assume that there are few predictor variables relative to the sample size. See Chapter 8 for advanced approaches and strategies that can deal with high-dimensional problems (more predictor variables than subjects). Also, the approach to modeling described in this chapter relies upon a subject matter expert. Here we usually mean a person (a physician) who knows a lot about the disease or condition in the target population and would like this statistical prediction model built. Hence, you yourself might be the subject matter expert.

4.1 Specifying the model type

By far the most important issue is to correctly specify the type of outcome variable. For each outcome variable, we will denote the standard regression method to be used to build a risk prediction model. If an alternative method is used, the results should either be compared to the results of the standard procedure or in some other way reveal a severe limitation of the standard procedure. For example, when Cox regression is the standard method and random forest for survival analysis is used instead, then the forest model should outperform the Cox regression model in terms of predictive performance. In other words, there is no reason to use a new, non-standard, method just for the sake of it. We fix the prediction time horizon and distinguish three often encountered cases: uncensored binary outcome, right-censored time-to-event outcome without competing risks, and right-censored time-to-event outcome with competing risks.

All settings require that all predictor variables are measured at a common time zero. With time-varying predictor variables, it would otherwise not be possible to predict risks for new subjects at the time origin because the predicted risk would depend on future values of the predictor variables.

4.1.1 Uncensored binary outcome

In the special case where the prediction time horizon equals the time origin, the model predicts the current status of the patients (diagnosis).

All patients are followed until the prediction time horizon, and thus it is known if the event has occurred or not in the time period between the time origin and the prediction time horizon. The main characteristic of this outcome setting is that the follow-up data of all subjects until the prediction time horizon are *uncensored*. Usually, the values of a binary outcome are coded as "1" (the event has occurred) or "0" (the event has not occurred). In uncensored data, competing risks may alter the interpretation of the event of interest but they are usually not a problem for the statistical analysis. The outcome status is known for subjects who experience a competing risk before the prediction time horizon ("0"): the event has not occurred and will never occur.

The standard method for building a model which predicts the risks of the outcome event is the *generalized linear regression model* with logistic regression featuring the logistic link function being by far the most popular special case. However, if they fit the data, two other link functions provide regression coefficients that have an easier interpretation. The log-link [154, 126, 127] leads to relative risks and the identity-link [93] to risk differences.

4.1.2 Right-censored time-to-event outcome (no competing risks)

Survival analysis is characterized by censored data. The most common form of censored data is called *right-censored* (Section 2.4.5). Some of the patients are lost to follow-up before the event of interest occurred. For those patients, it is only known that the event did not occur before the censoring time. The censoring time is the time at which the subject was last seen event-free. This observational pattern is very common in medical studies. It is referred to as *right censoring* because, on the timeline, the event time is then on the right of (i.e., greater than) the censoring time. Most statistical procedures rely on the assumption that a subject who is lost to follow-up will experience the event of interest at the same rate as the other subjects that are still followed up and will eventually experience the event if followed long enough. When there are predictor variables, such as subject and disease characteristics, this assumption can be relaxed to saying that subjects lost to follow-up are represented not by all other subjects, but by only those with similar predictor values. The standard method for building risk prediction models based on right-censored time-to-event data is Cox regression [47]. The partial likelihood [48] approach allows that the regression coefficients (hazard ratios) are estimated without a parameterization of the baseline hazard function. The baseline hazard function describes the hazard rate of the event where all predictor variables take the value zero. The baseline hazard function is usually not of interest. However, risk predictions from a Cox regression model depend on the hazard ratios and the baseline hazard function. Thus, in order to predict the risk of the outcome event at the prediction time horizon for a new subject, based on a Cox regression model, one has to estimate the baseline hazard function as well. The standard method for estimating the baseline hazard function is the Breslow estimator [33], a non-parametric estimator.

One should note that standard Cox regression requires that there are no competing risks. When there are competing risks, a naive application of Cox regression would lead to systematically too-high predicted risks very much in the same way as the Kaplan-Meier method would lead to systematically too-low survival probabilities [6]. This bias can be avoided either by adding a Cox regression model for the competing event to the equation [17, 135] or by switching to Fine-Gray regression; see Section 4.1.3.

For making a model that predicts the risks until a fixed prediction time horizon (Figure 2.1), subjects lost to follow-up after the time horizon are technically not censored as their event status at the prediction time horizon is known; these subjects are *event-free* at the prediction time horizon. It is possible and sometimes useful to artificially censor all event times that occur after the prediction time horizon (Section 7.6). The following example code shows 6 subjects of the oral cancer study for whom we have artificially censored the time-to-event outcome after 5 years (60 months) and for whom we have correspondingly reset the censoring status variable.

```
# R-code
oc$survtime.5years <- pmin(oc$survtime,60) # stop time after 5
    years
oc$survstatus.5years <- oc$survstatus # take a copy
oc[oc$survtime>60,]$survstatus.5years <- 0 # reset status
oc[,c("survtime","survstatus","survtime.5years","survstatus.5years"
    )]
```

survtime	survstatus	survtime.5years	survstatus.5years
29	1	29	1
100	1	60	0
91	1	60	0
109	0	60	0
6	1	6	1
69	0	60	0

All deaths that occur after 5 years are now censored. Application of the Cox regression model to the artificially censored time-to-event outcome yields the so-called stopped Cox regression model [179].

As alternatives to Cox regression, one can use the inverse probability of censoring weighting (IPCW) [39] or pseudo value regression [9] to estimate the t-year risk of the outcome event via a generalized linear regression model [55]. The IPCW approach may be less efficient than partial likelihood but has the benefit that it allows other link functions. Particularly, the log-link leads to risk ratios, the logit-link to odds ratios, and the identity-link to risk differences.

4.1.3   Right-censored time-to-event outcome with competing risks

In addition to the event of interest, other events can occur in the time period between the time origin and the prediction time horizon. A competing risk is an event after which the risk of the event of interest changes (Section 2.4.6). In the case where the competing risk is death, the risk of the event of interest is zero after the competing event has occurred. A competing risk can also be an event after which the event of interest is no longer of interest for other reasons.

The complication of the competing risk setting is due to right-censored data. For patients who are not lost to follow-up before the prediction time horizon, the status at the prediction time horizon is known: either the event of interest has occurred, or a competing risk has occurred, or the patient is event-free. However, for patients who are lost to follow-up before the prediction time horizon, it is only known that the event time is larger than the time at which the patient was last seen event-free; it remains unknown if the event of interest or a competing risk occurs first and if this happens before or after the prediction time horizon.

There are two standard methods for prediction in the situation with competing risks, and these are usually roughly equivalent in terms of prediction performance. The first is a combination of a series of cause-specific Cox regression models [17, 38, 135]. One has to specify a Cox regression model for the hazard rate of the event of interest and further Cox regression model(s) for the hazard rate(s) of the competing risk(s). The formula that obtains a predicted risk from a series of Cox regression models requires hazard ratios and baseline hazard functions for the event of interest and the competing risks [135].

The second approach is a class of direct regression models for the risk of the event of interest [159]. The most prominent choice is the negative log-log link which yields the Fine-Gray regression model [66]. However, the interpretation is enhanced with other link functions if they fit the data and predict reasonably well [73].

4.2   Benchmark model

Once the outcome type is set, one should compute the population average risk of the event at the prediction time horizon. A model which predicts the average risk to every patient is a model which is always available, i.e., it can be easily obtained in a given dataset, and it provides a useful benchmark for more complex models. Such a model ignores all predictor variables and is therefore referred to as the *null model*.

4.2.1   Uncensored binary outcome

In the uncensored binary outcome case, the null model predicts the outcome risk simply estimated by the number of events at the prediction time horizon divided by the number of subjects in the dataset. In the training dataset (n=174) of the in vitro fertilization study, in total 57 patients developed ovarian hyperstimulation syndrome, i.e., too many mature follicles. This happens as an adverse response to hormone treatment. Our null model thus predicts the risk of ovarian hyperstimulation syndrome mature follicles as $57/174 \approx 32.8\%$. We can obtain the null model by fitting a logistic regression model without predictor variables. This is useful for cross-validation. Note that the predicted risk is identical to the value 32.8% when the null model is applied, independent of the patient's characteristics.

```
# R-code
# logistic regression in learn data
nullmodel <- glm(ohss~1,data=ivftrain,family="binomial")
```

```
# predicted risk in test data
ivftest$risk.null <- predictRisk(nullmodel,newdata=ivftest)
# result does not depend on predictor variables
ivftest[1:5,c("cyclelen","bmi","age","smoking","ant.foll","risk.
    null")]
```

cyclelen	bmi	age	smoking	ant.foll	risk.null
28	24.98	32	Yes	5	0.3275862
30	26.26	25	Yes	13	0.3275862
32	19.94	36	No	30	0.3275862
29	20.28	37	No	22	0.3275862
31	32.77	30	No	25	0.3275862

4.2.2 Right-censored time-to-event outcome (without competing risks)

In the case with right-censored time-to-event outcome when there are no competing risks, we use the Kaplan-Meier estimator to obtain the benchmark model (null model).

The Kaplan-Meier method will be biased when there are competing risks or if the censoring mechanism depends on the predictor variables.

Specifically, at the prediction time horizon, we subtract the corresponding Kaplan-Meier estimate of survival from 100% to obtain the risk that the null model predicts for every subject.

In the training dataset of the oral cancer study [3], we can read off the predicted 10-year mortality risk from the Kaplan-Meier plot (Figure 4.1). The predicted 10-year mortality risk is 59.1%. The null model predicts a 59.1% risk of death to all subjects independent of the predictor values.

```
# R-code
library(riskRegression)
# Kaplan-Meier estimate in training set
km <- prodlim(Hist(survtime,survstatus)~1,data=octrain)
# Predicted risk at 5 and 10 years in test set
octest$km.risk5 <- round(100*predictRisk(km,newdata=octest,times
    =60),1)
octest$km.risk10 <- round(100*predictRisk(km,newdata=octest,times
    =120),1)
# Predicted risks do not depend on predictor variables
octest[1:5,c("age","gender","tobacco","tumorthickness","km.risk5","
    km.risk10")]
```

age	gender	tobacco	tumorthickness	km.risk5	km.risk10
62	Male	Ever	1.5	41.7	59.1
85	Female	Never	0.6	41.7	59.1
60	Male	Ever	1.3	41.7	59.1
65	Female	Never	0.3	41.7	59.1
39	Female	Never	0.3	41.7	59.1

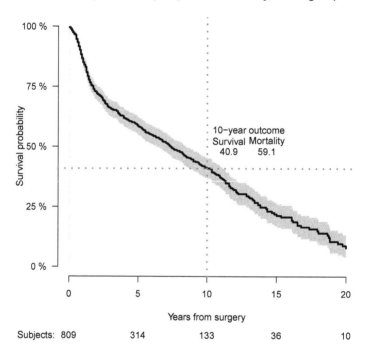

FIGURE 4.1
Kaplan-Meier estimate of the survival function in the training set of the oral cancer study.

4.2.3 Right-censored time-to-event with competing risks

In the case with competing risks, the null model is obtained with the Aalen-Johansen estimator [1]. In the active surveillance prostate cancer dataset [21] we apply the Aalen-Johansen method to estimate the absolute risk of cancer progression as a function of follow-up time since the cancer diagnosis.

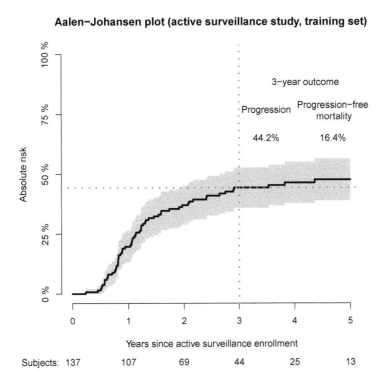

FIGURE 4.2
Aalen-Johansen estimate of the absolute risk (also called cumulative incidence) of cancer progression in the prostate cancer study.

The null model based on the Aalen-Johansen method predicts the 3-year risk of cancer progression as 44.2% (see Figure 4.2), thereby accounting for the competing risk of progression-free mortality. The predicted risk is 44.2% for all subjects independent of the predictor values. The Aalen-Johansen method applied to the competing event also shows that the 3-year risk of death without cancer progression is estimated as 16.4% in the training set. Thus, the overall probability of progression-free survival at the 3-year prediction time horizon is estimated at 39.4% (100.0 − 44.2 − 16.4 = 38.7).

```
# R-code
library(riskRegression)
# Aalen-Johansen estimate in training set
aj <- prodlim(Hist(asprogtime,asprog)~1,data=astrain)
# Predict the risks at 3 year horizon in the test set
astest$aj.progrisk3 <- round(100*predictRisk(aj,newdata=astest,
    times=3,cause="progression"),1)
astest$aj.deathrisk3 <- round(100*predictRisk(aj,newdata=astest,
    times=3,cause="death"),1)
# Predicted risks do not depend on predictor variables
astest[1:5,c("age5","psa","ct1","diaggs","aj.progrisk3","aj.
    deathrisk3")]
```

age5	psa	ct1	diaggs	aj.progrisk3	aj.deathrisk3
12.1	-3.0	cT1	3 and 3	44.2	16.4
11.0	-2.1	cT1	3 and 3	44.2	16.4
13.9	-3.1	cT2	3 and 3	44.2	16.4
13.9	-2.3	cT1	3 and 3	44.2	16.4
13.4	-3.1	cT1	3 and 3	44.2	16.4

4.3   Including predictor variables

The general aim of including variables in the prediction model is to increase the prediction performance of the model. This can only be achieved with predictor variables that are associated with the outcome of interest. For the sole purpose of making a prediction model, some will argue that a causal relationship between the predictor variable and the outcome is not required. For example, the effect of one of the predictor variables on the outcome variable could be (partly) mediated through other predictor variables. However, with a view toward the interpretation of the results of the prediction model in clinical practice, in particular, with respect to treatment decision, a causal interpretation of the model is something one should always aim for. In this work, we do not discuss this part of the modeling in detail but refer to the ongoing discussion on causal inference in the epidemiological and statistical literature [96].

4.3.1 Categorical predictor variables

Predictors with a finite number of possible values (categories) that cannot be sorted in a meaningful way are called nominal variables. Examples are gender, which defines two categories (female/male), and genotype, which defines three categories (AA, AB, BB). Nominal variables should be coded categorically and not numerically since any numeric coding for such a predictor would force the values into an arbitrary order.

Before including a categorical variable in the risk prediction model it is useful to count the number of patients in the dataset across the specified categories. Categories with few patients or few outcomes may need to be thoughtfully merged with other categories. Alternatively, if merging is not useful for subject matter reasons, patients in low-frequency categories can be omitted (but this changes the population in which the risk prediction model is applicable).

In the training set of the in vitro fertilization study, we fit a simple logistic regression model (simple = just one predictor variable) which predicts the risks of ovarian hyperstimulation syndrome based on smoking status.

```
# R-code
fit <- glm(ohss~smoking,data=ivftrain,family="binomial")
publish(fit,intercept=1)
```

The parameter estimates are the intercept (odds for non-smokers) and the odds ratio of smokers versus non-smokers (Table 4.1).

TABLE 4.1
In vitro fertilization study. Results of simple logistic regression show a borderline significant negative effect of smoking on the odds of treatment response in IVF training dataset.

Variable	Units	OddsRatio	CI.95	p-value
(Intercept)		0.595	[0.41;0.86]	0.006317
smoking	No	Ref		
	Yes	0.510	[0.25;1.05]	0.067062

Based on the simple logistic regression we can calculate a risk prediction model which predicts the risk of ovarian hyperstimulation syndrome conditional on smoking status (Figure 4.3). The formula of the risk prediction model is based solely on the odds ratios shown in Table 4.1 and given by 37.3% = expit(log(0.595)) for non-smokers and by 23.2% = expit(log(0.595 * 0.51)) for smokers, respectively.

```
# R-code
fit <- glm(ohss~smoking,data=ivftrain,family="binomial")
nd <- data.frame(smoking=c("No","Yes"))
nd$risk.ohss <- predictRisk(fit,newdata=nd)
```

nd

smoking	risk.ohss
No	0.3728814
Yes	0.2321429

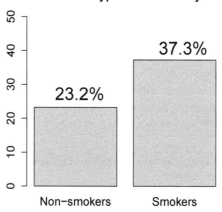

Risk of ovarian hyperstimulation syndrome

FIGURE 4.3
In vitro fertilization study. Simple logistic regression predicts the risk of ovarian hyperstimulation syndrome based on smoking status.

The risk of ovarian hyperstimulation syndrome is higher in non-smokers than in smokers, but for the interpretation of these results, one should keep in mind that smokers also have a lower chance of an appropriate response to the hormone treatment and, therefore, a lower chance of getting pregnant.

An ordinal predictor is a variable whose value takes a natural order. An example is disease stage in cancer ($I < II < III < IV$). Most often, ordinal predictors have to be treated as nominal, i.e., by ignoring the ordering. Forcing a linear effect upon the ordinal variable rarely yields an improvement of the predicted risks. For example, it is unlikely that the change of risk of relapse within 5 years between cancer disease stages I and II is exactly equal to the change between disease stages II and III and also exactly equal to the change between disease stages III and IV.

We consider the oral cancer data to illustrate the effect of including categorical variables in a prediction model for time-to-event outcome without competing risks. We fit a Cox regression model to predict 10-year overall mortality based on gender (nominal) and tumor grade (ordinal). The results are obtained with the following R-code and shown in Table 4.2.

```
# R-code
fit <- coxph(Surv(survtime, survstatus)~grade+gender,
        data=octrain,x=TRUE)
publish(fit)
```

TABLE 4.2
Oral cancer study. Results of Cox regression show significantly increased mortality hazard rates for grade "Moderate" and "Poor" compared to grade "Well." Gender does not seem to have a significant effect.

Variable	Units	HazardRatio	CI.95	p-value
grade	Well	Ref		
	Moderate	1.40	[1.09;1.81]	0.00852
	Poor	1.86	[1.34;2.56]	< 0.001
gender	Female	Ref		
	Male	1.08	[0.90;1.31]	0.40788

Based on the Cox regression model we extract the predicted mortality risk for the 10-year prediction time horizon in all possible combinations of gender and grade (see also Figure 4.4).

```
# R-code
fit <- coxph(Surv(survtime, survstatus)~grade+gender,
        data=octrain,x=1)
nd <- data.frame(expand.grid(grade=c("Well","Moderate","Poor"),
    gender=c("Male","Female")))
nd$risk.10years <- round(100*predictRisk(fit,
                times=120,newdata=nd),1)
nd
```

grade	gender	risk.10years
Well	Male	49.3
Moderate	Male	61.5
Poor	Male	71.7
Well	Female	46.6
Moderate	Female	58.6
Poor	Female	68.8

To illustrate the effect of categorical variables in the competing risk setting we consider the prostate cancer data. The Gleason score has 3 categories (GNA, 3 and 3, 3 and 4) and the clinical stage has two categories (cT1, cT2). We fit two cause-specific Cox regression models with two predictors (Gleason score and clinical stage) and no interaction terms, one model for cancer

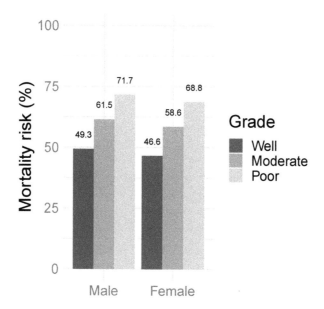

FIGURE 4.4
Oral cancer study. Cox regression predicts the 10-year mortality risk of oral
cancer patients based on grade and gender.

progression and one for progression-free mortality (Table 4.3). The table shows the hazard ratios for the Gleason score and clinical stage for the two models. We then predict the 3-year risk of cancer progression by combining the two cause-specific Cox regression models [18, 135]. The predicted 3-year risk for an individual depends on the effects (hazard ratios) that the predictor variables have on the two cause-specific hazard scales (c.f., Table 4.3) and the baseline hazard functions from each model. Note that a variable can have zero effect on the hazard rate of the event of interest, but still affect the absolute risk of the event of interest indirectly via an effect on the hazard rate of the competing risk (see also [124]). This makes sense, because increasing the risk of the event of interest must decrease the risk of the competing event, and vice versa, since one of the two events will ultimately occur given sufficient follow-up.

We also fit a Fine-Gray regression model (Table 4.4). The table shows the associations of the Gleason score and the clinical stage with the sub-distribution hazard rate. The association parameter is the sub-distribution hazard ratio, which does not have a nice interpretation [66]. However, there is a direct relationship between the sub-distribution hazard rate and the absolute risk of the event of interest.

```
# R-code
fit <- CSC(Hist(asprogtime,asprog)~diaggs+ct1,data=astrain)
publish(fit,diaggs="Gleason score",ct1="Clinical stage")
```

TABLE 4.3
Active surveillance prostate cancer study. Results of Cox regression analysis obtained in the training set. The table shows cause-specific hazard ratios with 95% confidence intervals for contrasts of the categorical variables Gleason score and clinical stage.

Variable	Units	Cancer progression	Progression-free mortality
Gleason score	GNA	Ref	Ref
	3 and 3	0.79 [0.35;1.77]	0.62 [0.24;1.62]
	3 and 4	1.65 [0.60;4.49]	0.26 [0.03;2.23]
Clinical stage	cT1	Ref	Ref
	cT2	1.87 [0.84;4.17]	1.39 [0.42;4.63]

We also predict the 3-year risk of cancer progression based on the Fine-Gray regression model shown in Table 4.4. Figure 4.5 shows the predicted risks in the six categories defined by all combinations of the Gleason score and the clinical stage; results obtained by combining the cause-specific Cox regression models (CSC, left panel) and based on the Fine-Gray regression model (FGR, right panel).

```
# R-code
fit <- FGR(Hist(asprogtime,asprog)~diaggs+ct1,data=astrain,
```

```
                cause="progression")
publish(fit)
```

TABLE 4.4
Active surveillance prostate cancer study. Results of Fine-Gray regression
analysis obtained in the training set. The table shows cause-specific sub-hazard
ratios with 95% confidence intervals for contrasts of the categorical variables
Gleason score and clinical stage.

Variable	Units	Sub-distribution hazard ratio
Gleason score	GNA	Reference
	3 and 3	0.83 [0.37;1.86]
	3 and 4	1.68 [0.65;4.32]
Clinical stage	cT2	Reference
	cT2	1.77 [0.75;4.21]

4.3.2 Continuous predictor variables

The linear predictor of a multiple regression model is the weighted sum
of the subject specific risk factors. The weights are the regression coef-
ficients, e.g., log-odds ratios or log-hazard ratios.

In most cases, continuous predictors should be kept continuous but without
necessarily forcing linear effects. In other words, just putting a continuous
predictor into a regression model will cause the resulting prediction model to
assume that each increment on the scale of the predictor will have a common
and constant effect on the linear predictor. The way in which these effects on
the linear predictor translate into effects on prediction risks is dependent on
the link function of the regression model.

In the in vitro fertilization study we fit a simple logistic regression model
which includes patient age as the only risk factor for ovarian hyperstimulation
syndrome.

```
# R-code
ivftrain$age5 <- ivftrain$age/5 # odds ratio per 5 year increase of
    age
fit <- glm(ohss~age5,data=ivftrain,family="binomial")
```

Figure 4.6 shows the resulting risk predictions for a given age when the
model forces a linear effect on the linear predictor. According to this model,
the risk is significantly decreasing with increasing age (per 5 years odds ra-
tio=0.63, CI_{95}=[0.40;0.99], p=0.047). On the log odds scale, this model assumes a linear relationship with age which, when translated to the absolute

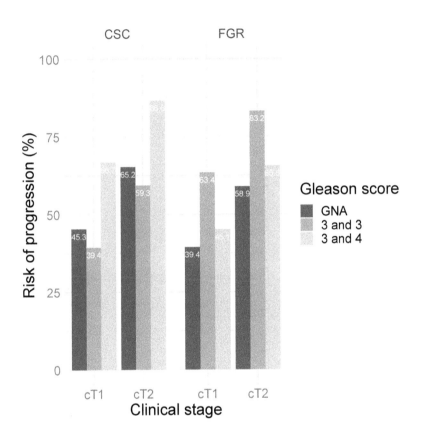

FIGURE 4.5
Active surveillance prostate cancer study. Predicted risks of cancer progression within 3 years after the start of an active surveillance program for all combinations of the two categorical variables. Results in panel CSC are based on the combined cause-specific Cox regression models (Table 4.3). The results in panel FGR are based on the Fine-Gray regression model (Table 4.4).

risks scale, shows a smoothly decreasing curve. The confidence bands illustrate
that the uncertainty is larger in regions of the age scale where our training
set contains little data.

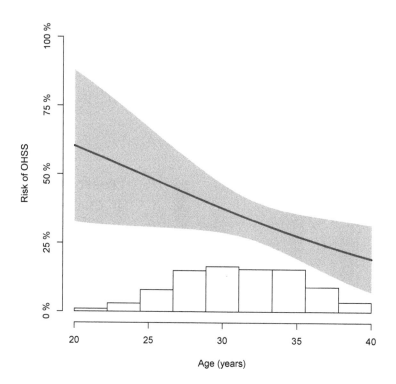

FIGURE 4.6
In vitro fertilization study. Predicted risk of ovarian hyperstimulation syndrome (OHSS) based on a simple logistic regression model which includes
patient age as the only predictor variable. The histogram shows the marginal
distribution of age in the training set.

However, the model shown in Figure 4.6 is tentatively misleading. Figure
4.7 shows the result of another logistic regression model also fitted to the
training set of the in vitro fertilization study.

```
# R-code
library(rms)
fit <- lrm(ohss~rcs(age),data=ivftrain)
```

This second model allows a non-linear effect of age which is estimated with a restricted cubic spline [87]. It indicates that the risk of ovarian hyperstimulation syndrome is low for young and old ages compared to middle age.

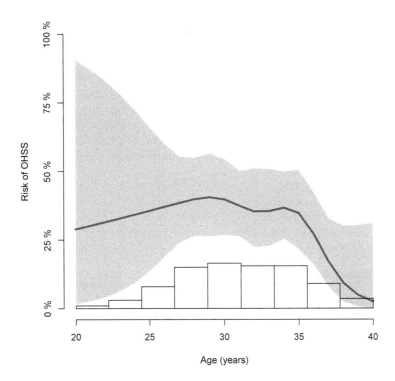

FIGURE 4.7
In vitro fertilization study. Predicted risk of ovarian hyperstimulation syndrome (OHSS) based on a logistic regression model which estimates a restricted cubic spline to describe a non-linear effect of patient age. The histogram shows the marginal distribution of age in the training set.

In the oral cancer dataset, a simple Cox regression model assumes a linear effect of tumor thickness on the hazard rate of all-cause mortality. The result is a significantly increasing hazard rate per increasing tumor thickness (hazard ratio= 1.52, CI_{95}= [1.40;1.66], $p < 0.001$). Due to the non-linear relationship between the hazard rate and the risk (risk = 1-survival probability), the effect on the 10-year risk is not linear (Figure 4.8).

```
# R-code
fit <-
```

```
coxph(Surv(survtime,survstatus)~tumorthickness,data=octrain,
    y=TRUE,x=TRUE)
```

Linear splines and restricted cubic splines [87] are two common options that could be explored to relax the linearity assumption. First note that a knot is any value in the range of a continuous variable. In the case of linear splines, the effect that the variable has on the outcome will potentially change at pre-selected knots. With restricted cubic splines the effect changes smoothly across most of the range of the predictor variable.

Splines have knots that must somehow be selected. Knot selection involves both the number of knots and the location of each knot. The two broad strategies for knot selection: one approach considers the outcome, and the other does not. When the knots are chosen without regard to the outcome, they typically are placed at various quantiles of the distribution of the predictor variable. When the outcome is considered, the placement should be driven by the prediction performance of the resulting risk prediction model.

For restricted cubic splines the number of knots matters. Typically, three knots are sufficient because the substantial part of a trend in a biological system is rarely multimodal.

```
# R-code
library(rms)
# fit Cox regression models
fit1=cph(Surv(survtime,survstatus)~tumorthickness,
    data=octrain,x=1,y=1)
# lsp means linear spline
fit2=cph(Surv(survtime,survstatus)~lsp(tumorthickness,c(.5,1,3)),
    data=octrain,x=1,y=1)
# rcs means restricted cubic spline
fit3=cph(Surv(survtime,survstatus)~rcs(tumorthickness,3),
    data=octrain,x=1,y=1)
# select tumor thickness values for which to predict
nd=data.frame(tumorthickness=c(0.1,.5,.75,seq(1,8,1)))
# extract 10 year predicted risks from Cox regression
R1=predictRisk(fit1, newdata=nd,times=120)
R2=predictRisk(fit2, newdata=nd,times=120)
R3=predictRisk(fit3, newdata=nd,times=120)
# put results in a table
nd$"10-year risk linear" <- 100*R1
nd$"10-year risk linear spline" <- 100*R2
nd$"10-year risk cubic spline" <- 100*R3
publish(nd,digits=1)
```

Table 4.5 and Figure 4.8 show predictions of 10-year all-cause mortality obtained with three different Cox regression models each making different

TABLE 4.5
For selected values of tumor thickness, 10-year mortality risk predictions of three Cox regression models. The first model assumes a linear effect on the linear predictor, the second uses a linear spline with three knots (0.5, 1, 3) and the third model uses restricted cubic splines with three knots selected by the software.

Tumorthickness	linear	linear spline	cubic spline
0.1	45.8	37.9	34.7
0.5	51.6	46.0	48.8
0.8	55.3	56.3	57.6
1.0	59.1	67.1	64.7
2.0	74.4	77.9	78.1
3.0	87.5	87.1	85.4
4.0	95.8	91.5	91.2
5.0	99.2	94.8	95.4
6.0	99.9	97.2	98.0
7.0	100.0	98.6	99.3
8.0	100.0	99.4	99.8

assumptions about the effect of tumor thickness on the hazard of all-cause mortality.

4.3.3 Interaction effects

In the context of multiple regression analysis, an interaction effect occurs when the effect of one variable depends on the value of another variable. Hence, in addition to outcome, there are at least two predictor variables involved in an interaction term. A better name for interaction is effect modification. The effect of one predictor variable is modified by another predictor variable. A higher-order interaction occurs when the effect of one variable on outcome depends on at least two other variables.

In the standard regression model framework, the specification of potential interaction effects should be determined prior to data analysis. In the usual scenario, the analyst is interviewing the subject matter expert for predictor variables, listening for the direction of effect. Occasionally, the expert will say that a particular predictor variable matters more or less in a particular subset of subjects defined by another predictor variable, suggesting an interaction term. These are the potential interaction terms that should be entered into the model. For the purpose of making a risk prediction model, it is most relevant to consider to what extent an interaction effect modifies the predicted risks. Obviously, including an interaction term in the regression model needs to be justified relative to the sample size.

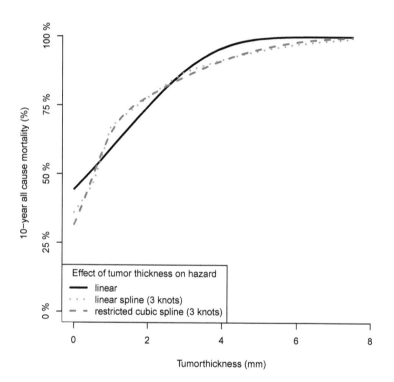

FIGURE 4.8
Oral cancer study. Linear and non-linear effects of tumorthickness on the linear predictor of a simple Cox regression model in the training data of the oral cancer study. Shown are the effects on the 10-year all-cause mortality.

In the prostate cancer study the following table shows 3-year predicted risks of cancer progression from a model which includes an interaction term. The effect of the PSA density (logarithmic scale, variable *psa*) is allowed to depend on the clinical stage (variable *ct1*). The cause-specific Cox regression models for progression and death are further adjusted for the Gleason score (variable *diaggs*):

```
# R-code
fit1 <- CSC(Hist(asprogtime,asprog)~psa+ct1+diaggs,data=astrain,
    cause="progression")
fit2 <- CSC(Hist(asprogtime,asprog)~psa*ct1+diaggs,data=astrain,
    cause="progression")
# select 12 examples
nd=expand.grid(diaggs=c("GNA","3 and 3","3 and 4"),
        ct1=c("cT1","cT2"),
        psa=c(-3,-1))
# predict 3-year risk of progression
R1 <- 100*predictRisk(fit1,newdata=nd,cause="progression",times=3)
R2 <- 100*predictRisk(fit2,newdata=nd,cause="progression",times=3)
cbind(nd,"No interaction term"=R1,"With interaction term"=R2)
```

TABLE 4.6
Active surveillance prostate cancer study. Predicted 3-year risks of progression by cause-specific Cox regression models for selected values of the Gleason score, clinical stage, and PSA density (logarithmic scale). The presence of the interaction term changes the predicted 3-year risks considerably for the last three examples but not very much for the first 9 examples.

Gleason score	Clinical stage	PSA (log)	3-year risk: No interaction term	3-year risk: With interaction term
GNA	cT1	−3.0	45.1	45.2
3 and 3	cT1	−3.0	40.2	40.1
3 and 4	cT1	−3.0	66.0	66.0
GNA	cT2	−3.0	62.7	61.7
3 and 3	cT2	−3.0	57.9	56.8
3 and 4	cT2	−3.0	84.2	83.3
GNA	cT1	−1.0	55.1	53.4
3 and 3	cT1	−1.0	50.1	48.7
3 and 4	cT1	−1.0	77.0	76.0
GNA	cT2	−1.0	72.6	84.5
3 and 3	cT2	−1.0	68.6	78.7
3 and 4	cT2	−1.0	91.6	95.8

In the selected 12 covariate values, the predicted 3-year risk of progression does change substantially for some of the examples (Table 4.6).

In the in vitro fertilization study, the effect of the number of antral follicles (considered as a continuous variable) on the risk of ovarian hyperstimulation syndrome could be modified by smoking status. Here we also adjust for age. Table 4.7 shows the predicted risks for six selected covariate patterns.

```
# R-code
fit1 <- glm(ohss~ant.foll+smoking+age,data=ivftrain,
        family="binomial")
fit2 <- glm(ohss~ant.foll*smoking+age,data=ivftrain,
        family="binomial")
# select 6 examples
nd <- expand.grid(ant.foll=c(10,30,50),
            age=c(30),
            smoking=factor(c("Yes","No")))
R1 <- 100*predictRisk(fit1,newdata=nd)
R2 <- 100*predictRisk(fit2,newdata=nd)
cbind(nd,"Without interaction term"=R1,"With interaction term"=R2)
```

TABLE 4.7
In vitro fertilization study. Predicted risks of ovarian hyperstimulation syndrome by two logistic regression models. The presence of the interaction term changes the predicted risks for all 6 examples.

Antral follicles	Age	Smoking	Without interaction term	With interaction term
10	30	Yes	5.1	1.6
30	30	Yes	48.9	59.4
50	30	Yes	94.5	99.2
10	30	No	12.5	16.3
30	30	No	71.8	66.3
50	30	No	97.8	95.2

4.4   Modeling strategy

4.4.1   Variable selection

We consider a list of the candidate predictor variables obtained from the subject matter expert (Section 2.4.2). We feel that obtaining this starting list from the expert and the literature is better than fishing for them by using the data. This is to avoid spurious associations with the outcome that will not be useful for predicting risks when faced with new patients. Also, the subject matter expert has a much better understanding of the underlying disease process. When we query the subject matter expert for the list of these candidate variables, it is important to note which of them are routinely collected and have a perceived direction of effect. So, the subject matter expert not only names a variable, but also defends that other medical centers measure this variable. This explains why the variable should matter when making a prediction by means of being routinely collected and having a direction of effect upon the outcome.

Once the outcome variable has been defined and the predictors identified, our strategy becomes easier to articulate. We first assume we are not in a situation where there are very few events or more predictor variables than subjects. Those situations require special care and are dealt with in Chapter 8. We will also not deal here with missing values, where imputation may be required. We do this in Section 7.5.

4.4.2 Conventional model strategy

With multiple predictor variables, there are many different multiple regression models that one can build by including effects of categorical and continuous predictor variables as well as interaction effects (Section 4.3). This is the case for all outcome types and logistic regression, Cox regression and Fine-Gray regression models. There are no genuine rules regarding how to build the best risk prediction model without asking the data (Section 4.4.3). And asking the data increases the risk of overfitting. Thus, when the aim is to use the data to find the best risk prediction model, cross-validation (Section 7.4) is an indispensable tool. In order to assess a particular risk prediction model obtained with any of the available modeling algorithms (Section 8), benchmarking is very important.

The null model benchmark (Section 4.2) is needed to separate the wheat from the chaff; all risk prediction models have to be better than that. For the interpretation of the prediction performance of a particular model, usually more work is needed. A very useful concept for the experimental part of modeling is to establish another benchmark that does make use of the predictor variables. Thus, the modeling process begins with the specification of a conventional model (see also Section 2.6.1). The conventional model contains the basic set of predictors that virtually anyone familiar with the subject matter would expect to see in the model. Moreover, no data-dependent modeling steps are applied to identify this model. The goal of any experimental model is to outperform the null by a larger degree than does the conventional model. In some cases, the conventional model is being used in clinical practice today. Any experimental model needs to outperform that model. Moreover, any experimental model needs to outperform a re-fitted conventional model with regression coefficients specific to our training dataset. In Chapter 6 we illustrate the conventional model strategy by applying it to real data.

4.4.3   Whether to use a standard regression model or something else

Many different statistical methods are available nowadays to help build a prediction model. Commonly applied methods are either based on regression analysis and testing of associations, or use a Bayesian approach, or purely data-based machine learning. Whatever the methods are, there will always be personal preferences and data-dependent decisions involved during the often long process from the raw dataset to the final prediction model. Since all modeling strategies are personal, in the sense that researchers have different preferences at different stages of the modeling process, it is not constructive to provide an exhaustive survey. Instead, we start by noting that for practical purposes it is often reasonable to expect that all sound strategies when applied to the same dataset should end up with comparable results: the predicted risk of any new patient should not change dramatically when we switch between models built with two equally sophisticated modeling algorithms.

However, it is important to recognize that not all commonly applied strategies are sound, and unfortunately, erroneous results frequently pass the barrier of peer review. In order to be able to catch problems in the modeling strategy at an early stage, such as systematic overfitting of the data, it is necessary that all data-dependent and data-independent steps of modeling are collected in a computer algorithm. The algorithm should produce the final risk prediction model when it is applied to a learning set of data. The applicability of all modeling steps through a computer algorithm is a requirement for all internal validation designs which rely on repeated splits of the data into learning and validation part [58, 32].

When thinking about the modeling strategy and the many alternatives available, the role of cross-validation becomes critical (Section 7.4). Any time the modeler produces a model and then changes something to look at the impact on performance, the need for another layer of cross-validation is triggered (Chapter 8). This is needed to avoid overfitting the training data. Because, when modeling decisions are based on the training data, then the model will predict especially well in the training data. This includes seemingly harmless decisions such as whether to include or remove one of the predictor variables, or whether to log-transform a continuous predictor variable.

Each strategy should be fully specified and result in a single prediction model when fitted to data. In other words, all modeling decisions should be made prior to the examination of model performance. If various settings are changed (also known as tuning parameters) and multiple models compared, this will artificially make the prediction technique appear to perform better than it does. This is like a stable that enters multiple horses into a race prior to stable evaluation. The typical example of this is when various settings of something like an artificial neural network are varied, and several of those models are compared with logistic regression. One combination of settings seems to do better than the logistic regression model. Those settings should have been determined prior to the comparison with logistic regression and independent of the relationship between predictors and outcome in the dataset at hand (i.e., blinded to outcome).

4.5 Advanced topics

4.5.1 How to prevent overfitting the data

In small samples, even pre-specified regression models tend to overfit the data and this leads to overstated effects. An overfit model weights the predictors too much. Shrinkage is a method which reduces these overstated effects and aims to improve prediction performance [89]. Essentially, the beta coefficients move closer to zero with shrinkage (Section 8.2.1). This in turn means that individualized predicted risks move closer to the prevalence (See Figure 8.4).

In the in vitro fertilization data, we illustrate the effect of shrinkage by comparing an unshrunk logistic regression model with two other logistic regression models that are shrunk with different degrees of penalty. All three models use restricted cubic splines for the effects of age, cycle length, and the number of antral follicles, and they further adjust for smoking. Table 4.8 shows the predicted risks of ovarian hyperstimulation syndrome for selected covariate patterns.

```
# R-code
library(rms)
fit1 <-lrm(ohss~rcs(ant.foll,3)+rcs(age,3)+rcs(cyclelen,3)+smoking,
       data=ivftrain)
fit2 <-lrm(ohss~rcs(ant.foll,3)+rcs(age,3)+rcs(cyclelen,3)+smoking,
       data=ivftrain, penalty=5)
fit3 <-lrm(ohss~rcs(ant.foll,3)+rcs(age,3)+rcs(cyclelen,3)+smoking,
       data=ivftrain,penalty=10)
# select 5 covariate patterns
nd=expand.grid(ant.foll=c(10,20), age=28,
          cyclelen=c(27,32), smoking="No")
# predict risks
R1=100*predictRisk(fit1,nd)
R2=100*predictRisk(fit2,nd)
R3=100*predictRisk(fit3,nd)
cbind(nd,"no penalty"=R1,"penalty 5"=R2,"penalty 10"=R3)
```

Note that indeed the predicted risks move towards the prevalence as the penalty increases. In Section 8.2.1 we explain that cross-validation should be used to determine the "right" amount of penalty.

TABLE 4.8
In vitro fertilization study. Predicted risks of ovarian hyperstimulation syndrome by three logistic regression models with varying penalty to correct for overfitting.

Antral follicles	Age	Cycle length	Smoking	No penalty	Penalty 5	Penalty 10
10	28	27	No	5.0	15.8	17.9
20	28	27	No	36.4	32.3	31.7
10	28	32	No	9.2	26.2	29.2
20	28	32	No	52.2	47.4	46.8

Shrinkage is particularly useful when the number of predictor variables is large relative to the number of subjects in the dataset.

Another benefit of shrinkage is to allow the use of more predictors than would otherwise have been acceptable, even to the point of having more predictors than subjects. The most common form of shrinkage is called ridge regression. With ridge regression, you must choose a penalty value to control how much shrinkage is applied. Because shrinkage is a double-edged sword, the degree to which one shrinks needs to be optimized. Obviously, shrinking the beta coefficients too far will at some point result in a reduction in predictive performance. Therefore, we recommend cross-validation to optimize the shrinkage penalty parameter. Note that this internal cross-validation will require the need for outer cross-validation to validly evaluate the entire process of model building. Also, you need to verify that the final model results do not vary with the random seed used to determine in which way the data are split during cross-validation, such as repeatedly varying the seed.

4.5.2   How to deal with missing values

If a predictor variable has many missing values, that likely indicates that the variable is not routinely collected in practice. Thus, omitting that predictor may be a sensible thing to do. If a predictor is not extensively missing and it is believed to be important for the prediction performance, a strategy for handling missing values can be used (Section 7.5). The most commonly used and accepted approach seems to be multiple imputation. While counter-intuitive, missing values in predictors should be imputed with knowledge of the outcome [16]. In any case, it is necessary to integrate the handling of missing data into the modeling algorithm somehow. Further, some advice is needed for how to use a risk prediction model when the future patient cannot provide values for all predictor variables for one reason or another (Section 7.5.2).

4.5.3 How to deal with non-converging models

In this case, your model is too complex given the data that you have. This may be due to sample size, number of predictors, missing values in the predictors, too many knots used for splines, or use of rare categories.

We can easily construct this phenomenon. For example, using the training data of the oral cancer study, the following model has too many interaction terms.

```
# R-code
fit <-coxph(Surv(survtime,survstatus)~tumorthickness + age + gender
   * race * tobacco * site,
       data=octrain,y=TRUE,x=TRUE)
```

```
Warning message:
In fitter(X, Y, strats, offset, init, control, weights = weights,  :
  Loglik converged before variable  13,22,33,39,41,42,43,44,45,49,54,56;
  coefficient may be infinite.
```

Problems arise with standard regression models (logistic regression, Cox regression) when there are categorical variables where some categories have zero or 100% events. There are several solutions. You might be able to merge rare categories to achieve categories with a mixture of outcomes. You could also omit predictors or reduce the number of knots in the splines. Shrinkage alone can often solve your convergence problem. Indeed, with ridge regression, you can include more predictor variables than subjects (Section 8.2.1).

4.6 What you should put in your manuscript

4.6.1 Baseline tables

Baseline tables show the distributions of the predictor variables. For continuous predictor variables we can choose between median (IQR=inter quartile range) and mean (SD=standard deviation) but could also show the range. The tables can show that gender is similar across centers, for example, but adding p-values here is rather useless. Baseline tables should show the number of missing values. See Table 4.9 for an example.

```
# R-code
tab1 <- summary(utable(gender~age+deep.invasion+tobacco+
    tumorthickness+grade,
              data=octrain,
              summary.format="median(x) (IQR(x)) [range(x)]"),
          show.pvalue=0)
tab1
```

TABLE 4.9

Oral cancer study. An example of descriptive statistics and missing value counts for a baseline table using the training set. The predictor variables summarized in the table are all measured at the time origin (baseline).

Variable	Level	Female (n=357)	Male (n=441)	Total (n=798)
age	median (IQR) [range]	64 (21) [17, 88]	60 (18) [18, 87]	62 (20) [17, 88]
deep.invasion	No	282 (82.7)	344 (80.9)	626 (81.7)
	Yes	59 (17.3)	81 (19.1)	140 (18.3)
	missing	16	16	32
tobacco	Ever	199 (56.1)	348 (78.9)	547 (68.7)
	Never	156 (43.9)	93 (21.1)	249 (31.3)
	missing	2	0	2
tumorthickness	median (IQR) [range]	0.7 (0.8) [0.0, 7.5]	0.8 (0.9) [0, 5]	0.8 (0.9) [0.0, 7.5]
grade	Well	77 (21.6)	84 (19.0)	161 (20.2)
	Moderate	231 (64.7)	290 (65.8)	521 (65.3)
	Poor	49 (13.7)	67 (15.2)	116 (14.5)

In case of a one-time split of the data (Section 7.4.1), a baseline table may compare training with the validation set. See Table 4.10 for an example.

```
# R-code
ivf$set <- factor(ivf$train,levels=c(TRUE,FALSE),
        labels=c("Training","Validation"))
tab1 <- summary(utable(set~Q(age)+cyclelen+Q(bmi)+fsh+ant.foll+
    smoking,data=ivf),
        show.pvalues=0)
tab1
```

4.6.2 Follow-up tables

Follow-up tables show the distribution of predictor variables conditional on the event status at the prediction time horizon. When the event status is uncensored for all subjects at the prediction time horizon, this seems to be straightforward. When the outcome is a right-censored time-to-event variable, this is not straightforward. First one needs to select a prediction time horizon. In the situation without competing risks there are three groups of patients for any given prediction time horizon: event, event-free, unknown (i.e., right-censored before horizon). With competing risks, there are four (or

TABLE 4.10
In vitro fertilization study. Example baseline table comparing training and validation splits of the in vitro fertilization data.

Variable	Level	Training (n=174)	Validation (n=102)	Total (n=276)
age	median [iqr]	32.5 [30, 35]	33 [31, 36]	33 [30, 35]
cyclelen	mean (sd)	28.5 (2.1)	28.5 (2.1)	28.5 (2.1)
bmi	median [iqr]	22.1 [20.4, 24.1]	22.5 [20.5, 24.3]	22.2 [20.4, 24.2]
fsh	mean (sd)	6.6 (1.7)	6.6 (1.9)	6.6 (1.7)
ant.foll	mean (sd)	20.2 (9.2)	19.9 (8.3)	20.1 (8.9)
smoking	No	118 (67.8)	67 (65.7)	185 (67.0)
	Yes	56 (32.2)	35 (34.3)	91 (33.0)

more) possibilities. Table 4.11 shows a 5-year follow-up table training set of the prostate cancer active surveillance study.

```
# R-code
tab2 <- followupTable(Hist(asprogtime,asprog)~age+ct1+erg.status,
    data=as,followup.time=5)
tab2
```

4.6.3 Regression tables

In this chapter, we have provided several examples of regression tables showing odds ratios and hazard ratios. We have explained in Section 2.7.3 that these parameters do not have a direct interpretation in terms of prediction performance. To illustrate this limitation further in the case of the Cox regression model we note an alternative interpretation of the hazard ratios [50]. Table 4.12 shows a simple transformation of the hazard ratios into probabilistic indices [50]. For example, this allows the following conclusion sentence. The probability of surviving longer with a grade "Moderate" than with a grade "Well" is significantly below 50% (probabilistic index: 42.71%) for given values of the other predictor variables. This interpretation demonstrates that the hazard ratio is a rank statistic with information regarding the expected order of the event times.

```
# R-code
fit <- coxph(Surv(survtime,survstatus)~age+gender+tumorthickness+
    grade,data=octrain)
```

TABLE 4.11
Active surveillance prostate cancer study. Example of a follow-up table with
descriptive statistics for each outcome status at the 5-year prediction time
horizon. The column "Unknown" contains data from subjects lost to follow-
up (right-censored) before the 5-year prediction time horizon.

Variable	Outcome 5 years after start of active surveillance			
	Progression (n=102)	Death (n=50)	Unknown (n=45)	Event-free (n=20)
Age, mean (sd)	65.3(3.4)	65.5(4.5)	65.4(3.2)	63.8(3.6)
CT1	87(85.3)	47(94.0)	43(95.6)	20(100.0)
CT2	15(14.7)	3(6.0)	2(4.4)	0(0.0)
ERG negative	39(38.2)	34(68.0)	34(75.6)	14(70.0)
ERG positive	63(61.8)	16(32.0)	11(24.4)	6(30.0)

```
publish(fit,probindex=TRUE)
```

Also, it is possible to fit an absolute risk regression model where the regression coefficients are ratios of absolute risks with an interpretation relative
to a prediction time horizon [73]. Using our prostate cancer study for illustration, Table 4.13 shows absolute risk ratios (ARR) at the 5-year prediction
time horizon based on a regression model fitted to the 5-year event status using inverse probability weights to deal with right censoring. According to this
model and given values for the other predictor variables, ERG status positive
patients have an 80% increased risk of relapse within 5 years from baseline:
the absolute 5-year risk ratio has the value 1.8.

```
# R-code
fit <- ARR(Hist(asprogtime, asprog)~ct1+erg.status+age5+psa+ppb5+
    lmax,
        data=astrain, times=5, cause="progression")
publish(fit)
```

Factor	ARR	CI$_{95}$	p-value
ct1cT2	0.93	[0.6;1.4]	0.739
erg.statusPositive	1.8	[1.3;2.7]	0.001
age5	0.97	[0.8;1.2]	0.775
psa	1.2	[1.0;1.5]	0.029
ppb5	1.02	[1.0;1.1]	0.548
lmax	1.10	[1.0;1.3]	0.177

TABLE 4.12
Oral cancer study. Example of a table showing the results of a Cox regression model where we use the probabilistic index instead of the hazard ratio. The probabilistic index is a simple transformation of the hazard ratio with a more intuitive interpretation. For example, the probability that a patient who is one year older than an otherwise similar patient (same gender, tumorthickness and grade) has the event earlier is 49.2%.

Variable	Units	ProbIndex	CI.95	p-value
age		49.2	[49.0;49.4]	< 0.001
gender	Female	Ref		
	Male	48.8	[44.1;53.6]	0.6373
tumorthickness		40.2	[38.1;42.4]	< 0.001
grade	Well	Ref		
	Moderate	42.7	[36.6;49.0]	0.0242
	Poor	42.1	[34.1;50.5]	0.0637

TABLE 4.13
Active surveillance prostate cancer study. Example of a regression table showing absolute risk ratios at the 5-year prediction time horizon. According to this model, a one-unit increase of baseline PSA increases the absolute 5-year risk of progression by a factor of 1.2.

FACTOR	ARR	CI$_{95}$	p-value
ct1cT2	0.93	[0.6;1.4]	0.739
erg.statusPositive	1.8	[1.3;2.7]	0.001
age5	0.97	[0.8;1.2]	0.775
psa	1.2	[1.0;1.5]	¡0.029
ppb5	1.02	[1.0;1.1]	0.548
lmax	1.10	[1.0;1.3]	0.177

4.6.4   Risk plots

To illustrate the results of a medical risk prediction model, it is sometimes useful to show the impact of a single predictor variable on the risk of the event. In standard regression models, the change in predicted risk triggered by a change of a single predictor variable depends on the values of the other predictor variables. In logistic regression models, it further depends on the intercept, and in Cox regression models, it further depends on the baseline hazard function. Thus, in order to visualize the effect of a single predictor variable on the risk scale, we need to choose specific values. It is common to select means or medians for these values, yet this combination may not be prevalent in the data or even in the population. Still, this may give a nice view of the shape of the effect. Panel A of Figure 4.9 shows the effect of the number of antral follicles on the risk of ovarian hyperstimulation syndrome for given values of the other predictor variables based on a multiple logistic regression model which uses a restricted cubic spline to model the effect of the number of antral follicles. The other continuous variables (age, cycle length, BMI, FSH) have additive and linear effects on the linear predictor (Section 2.5.5) of the model.

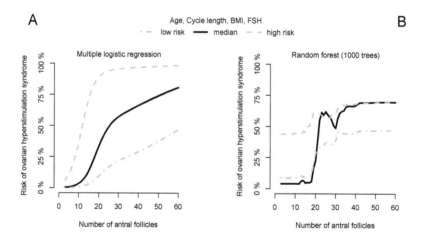

FIGURE 4.9

In vitro fertilization study. The impact of the number of antral follicles on the risk of ovarian hyperstimulation syndrome in a multiple logistic regression (Panel A) and a random forest model (Panel B) both adjusted for age, cycle length, BMI and FSH. The black line represents median values for the other predictors in the model, the light blue line and the orange line correspond to those values of the other predictors associated with the minimum and maximum risks, respectively.

Similar risk plots can be obtained with any machine learning approach to risk prediction modeling (Chapter 8). For example, a random forest (Section 8.3.1) allows non-linear relationships for all continuous predictor variables and higher-order interactions. Panel B of Figure 4.9 shows the effect of the number of antral follicles on the risk of ovarian hyperstimulation syndrome for given values of the other predictor variables based on a random forest with 1000 trees. We see that the predicted risks of the forest are less extreme compared to the logistic regression. The fact that the light blue line crosses the black line illustrates that the forest can potentially pick up complex interactions. We also see that the predictions of the random forest are not monotone functions of the number of antral follicles. This behavior where small changes of a variable can let the predicted risks jump up and down would clearly hamper the application of the random forest model in clinical practice.

When there are only two continuous predictor variables, a risk-level plot is an interesting option to illustrate a medical risk prediction model. Figure 4.10 shows risk prediction models based on logistic regression and random forests, respectively, each using the continuous predictor variables antral follicle count and age of our in vitro fertilization study to predict the risk of ovarian hyperstimulation syndrome. The logistic regression model uses a restricted cubic spline for the effect of the antral follicle count. We also see that the risk is decreasing with increasing age. The random forest model shows a risk mosaic where the predicted risk at any point in the plane reflects the average outcome of the training data in a neighborhood around the point (Section 8.3.1).

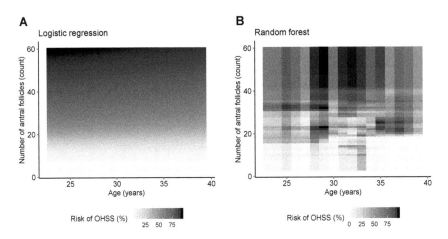

FIGURE 4.10
In vitro fertilization study. Risk-level plots for risk prediction models based on logistic regression (Panel A) and random forest (Panel B) and two continuous predictors of the training set. The color represents the risk of ovarian hyperstimulation syndrome.

Similar risk plots can be obtained from a Cox regression model or Fine-Gray regression model after first specifying a single prediction time horizon. When the outcome is a time-to-event variable, however, the predicted risks of a model can also be visualized for varying prediction time horizons. Figure 4.11 shows the predicted all-cause mortality risk of a Cox regression model as a function of time for best, average and worst-case scenarios defined by the extreme values of the predictor variables.

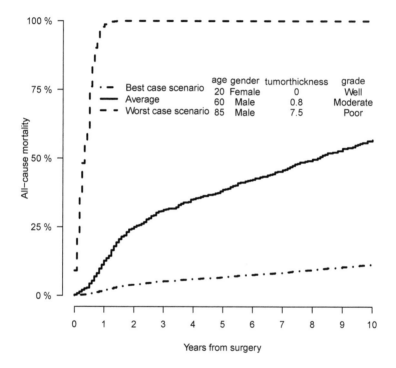

FIGURE 4.11
Oral cancer study. All-cause mortality risks predicted by Cox regression using predictor variables age, gender, tumorthickness, and grade.

4.6.5   Nomograms

Prediction models derived from regression models are often presented in tables showing odds ratios or hazard ratios. When the model includes regression splines or interactions between predictor variables, or both, such tables become increasingly difficult to read and comprehend. Generally, presenting the impact of the predictor variables on the risk scale would be more interpretable. Nomograms are graphical depictions of risk prediction models using scales with points. The user draws lines to assign points, sums the points to arrive at a total, and then draws another line to determine predicted probability from the total. For risk prediction models derived from logistic regression, nomograms are easily produced. Figure 4.12 shows an example based on the data of our in vitro fertilization study where we fit a logistic regression model with additive effects of age (linear), antral follicle count (restricted cubic spline) and smoking status (yes/no).

The attraction of a nomogram display is that it easily illustrates predicted risks from models with several predictors. Nomograms take unfriendly coefficients produced by a statistical software package and re-scales them on a friendly, usually 100-point, scale. In other words, the axes on the nomogram come from the coefficients determined through statistical analysis. When needing to convey a risk prediction model on a piece of paper, nomograms are a very attractive choice. Of particular note is that nomograms can display nonlinear effects as well as interaction effects, which are harder to put into tables.

```
# R-code
uu <- datadist(ivf)
options(datadist="uu")
fit <- lrm(ohss~age+rcs(ant.foll)+smoking,data=ivf)
plot(nomogram(fit,fun=function(x)1/(1+exp(-x)),   # or fun=plogis
           funlabel=paste0("Risk of OHSS")))
```

For risk prediction models derived from Cox regression, one needs to pick one or more prediction time horizons. Figure 4.13 shows a nomogram of a Cox regression model fitted to the data of the oral cancer study where an interaction term is used.

```
# R-code
u <- datadist(octrain)
options(datadist="u")
fit <- cph(Surv(survtime,survstatus)~age*grade+gender+rcs(
    tumorthickness),
        data=octrain,
        surv=1)
surv <- Survival(fit)
nom <- nomogram(fit, fun=list(function(x) 1-surv(60, x),
                  function(x) 1-surv(120, x)),
        funlabel=c("5-year risk",
                "10-year risk"))
plot(nom, xfrac=.5)
```

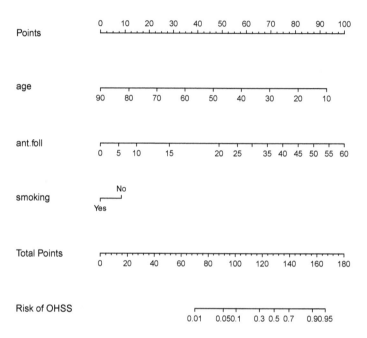

FIGURE 4.12

In vitro fertilization study. The nomogram should be read as follows. You first find the patient's age on the "age" axis and draw a line straight up to the Points axis to see how many points she gets for her age. For example, if she is 30 years old, she gets about 70 points. Next, do the same for the "ant.foll" axis. For a value of 15, she gets another 28 points. This process is repeated for each predictor, and the total points are summed. Her total points are then located on the Total Points axis, and a line is drawn straight down to get her risk of OHSS. For total points of 120, the risk is about 35%.

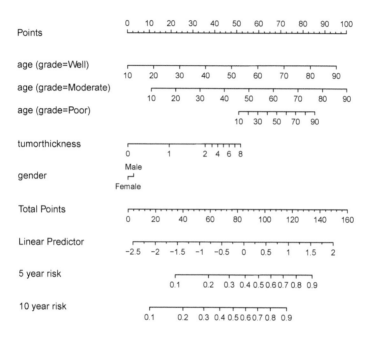

FIGURE 4.13

Oral cancer study. Nomogram illustrating an interaction between age and grade, with two prediction horizons. To use, first find the axis corresponding to the patient's grade, then find how many points he gets for his age. Next, move to the tumorthickness axis and work down. After calculating the patient's total points, draw a line straight down through both prediction horizon axes to determine his or her 5- and 10-year risks.

4.7   Deployment

4.7.1   Risk charts

When there are only a few predictor variables involved it is sometimes possible to show all possible risk predictions in a color chart, such as the European high-risk charts for 10-year risks of fatal cardiovascular disease [145]. However, this is really restricted to at most two continuous predictor variables. More complex situations require a full-blown Internet risk calculator.

4.7.2   Internet calculator

Free online applications seem to be the preferred route for risk prediction model dissemination. Software can do error checking, all necessary computations, including possible imputation, very quickly. Trumped only by embedding prediction models into the electronic health record, where the models would be executed automatically with no extra clinician effort, Internet risk calculators are proliferating. One site with many calculators is http://rcalc.ccf.org. This site runs R on a shiny server hosted by Amazon Web Services. This sophistication allows us to deploy machine learning models such as those based on random forests.

4.7.3   Cost-benefit analysis (waiting lists)

Generally, the utility of a risk prediction depends on the clinical context. In some settings, decisions have to be made regarding who to test or who to treat (first). An example is a waiting list for organ donation. Another example is the recent coronavirus pandemic where many health care systems did not have sufficient capacity for diagnostic testing and (sadly) for treatment [35, 161]. In such cases, a risk prediction model can be applied on everyone in the waiting list, e.g., in order to identify the subjects who would benefit most from the transplant, or are most likely to test COVID-19 positive.

The result is a ranking of persons according to their need. Figure 4.14 shows the tradeoffs of avoiding negative tests versus missing positive cases. Using a risk prediction model and a low cut-off, for example 1.5%, as a trigger to order testing will allow us to continue to identify the vast majority of COVID positive cases (assuming we maintain our other selection criteria for testing and add this additional requirement) while being able to avoid testing a large proportion of patients who are indeed COVID negative. This may be appropriate in a situation where testing supplies are abundant and one wants to get a comprehensive survey of the present extent of COVID-19 in the population. Conversely, in a resource-limited setting (e.g., hospital facing a surge), a cut-off greater than 1.5% or more may be more appropriate, in order to optimize the chance of avoiding unnecessary testing.

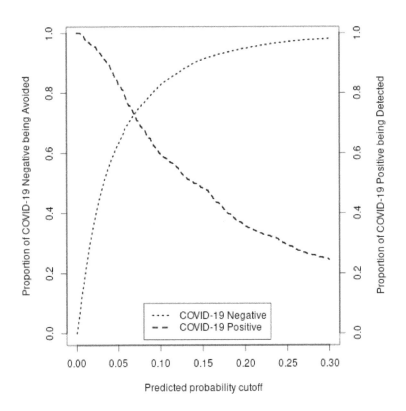

FIGURE 4.14

Proportion of COVID-19 (-) tests being avoided (dotted line) versus proportion of COVID-19 (+) tests being identified (dashed line) at different predicted probability cut-offs. For example, if a predicted probability of 0.25 and beyond was required before testing, nearly all negative cases would have been avoided, but about 70% of positive cases would have been missed.

When one can only afford to test or treat 17 persons, the calculus is simple: choose the top 17 from the ranked waiting list (in decreasing order of the predicted benefit). Of course, rival risk prediction models may produce different rankings, and it may be of interest to analyze the agreement of several rankings [61].

5

Does my model predict accurately?

In this chapter, we assume that a risk prediction model has been built which predicts event probabilities. For a single individual, the model provides the risk that the event of interest is present or will occur between the time origin and the prediction time horizon. The predictions are based on individual characteristics measured or evaluated at the time origin. Here we introduce and explain the concepts and statistical tools for assessing the prediction performance of a single risk prediction model. Chapter 6 uses the same concepts to compare risk prediction models and to assess the added value of a predictor variable. See Chapters 4 and 8 for algorithms that build risk prediction models.

The aim is now to assess how well the model predicts for new patients. The following applies whether internal cross-validation or external validation is performed (Section 2.6.2). But, to quantify the prediction performance of the model in new patients, one of the two validation procedures should be used in order to avoid overfitting bias – which naturally occurs when the model's performance is estimated on its learning data. With external validation, the prediction model is fitted with a training dataset, and the performance metrics and graphs are calculated with a test dataset. With internal cross-validation, the one and only purpose dataset is randomly split into training data and test datasets. This is repeated sufficiently many times, and performance metrics and graphs are calculated as averages across the splits.

For the sole purpose of illustration, in this chapter, we split our example datasets only once and train models on 63% of the data and then calculate performance measures in the remaining 37% of the data. A single split of the purpose dataset is not recommended in most real applications for efficiency reasons (the model trained in the full data should outperform the model trained in a reduced training set) and because the results of a single random split may depend grossly on the random seed, i.e., the results would be different when the data were split in a different way. We recommend the work of Faraway, who discusses this topic in depth, and writes, "If it becomes clear that there is insufficient data in the split datasets to find and estimate a model, then the analyst can always revert to the full data approach (but a switch from full to split cannot be allowed)" [64]. See Section 7.4 for more details and better alternatives to the single-split approach.

We address the three different settings that correspond to the three outcome types: uncensored binary, right-censored without competing risks, and right-censored with competing risks. With uncensored binary outcome at the prediction time horizon, all subjects in the dataset are in one of two possible states: either the event has occurred or it has not. In the uncensored binary setting there can be competing risks, for example death without the event, and then subjects in the "no event" state are in fact a mixture of those who experienced the competing risks before the prediction horizon and those alive and event-free at the prediction time horizon. In the right-censored survival setting at the prediction time horizon, the outcome is still binary; the event has occurred or not, but there is the possibility that the outcome is not known because the subject was not followed until the prediction time horizon (right-censored). The third setting deals with competing risks and censored data at the same time. At the prediction time horizon, all subjects are in one of three possible states: the event has occurred, a competing risk has occurred, or the subject is event-free. Due to early end of follow-up (censored observation), for some subjects, the state at the prediction time horizon is not observed (see also Section 4.6.2). See Section 2.7.4 for further discussion of censored data versus competing risks.

5.1 Model assessment roadmap

Here we describe three basic activities that are recommended. These are suggested, regardless of the event type (e.g., binary or survival). Note that these activities generally look at performance across a sample of data and do not necessarily allow a personalized interpretation. However, these activities can be applied to subsets of patients (just not individual ones) to see if performance varies across subsets of the data or along with a specific predictor variable. Moreover, these approaches are used to evaluate the performance of a model in isolation. In Chapter 6, we describe techniques to compare rival models.

5.1.1 Visualization of the predictions

To begin, apply the model to the subjects in the validation data by using the prediction time horizon and save the predicted risks. Next, calculate simple summary statistics, like the mean, median and range of the predicted risks. Then, visualize the subject-specific predicted risks. This seems like a very simple activity, yet it can reveal some important aspects of the model. Consider a simple histogram of the predicted probabilities obtained when the model is applied to the validation data. Are the predicted probabilities mostly concentrated in a very narrow region, say around the average of the predicted risks? If so, the model is not making very extreme predictions. This suggests that the model may not be highly discriminating since most of the patients will have very similar predictions. Are there a few outliers, i.e., some patients with extreme predictions away from the bulk of the predictions? If so, those observations should be investigated, particularly with respect to errors in the data.

Next, consider plotting the predicted risks broken down by subgroups of the predictors. Do the men and women in the validation data have very different predictions? This can be visualized using boxplots. For a continuous predictor variable, a scatterplot can be shown with the scale of the variable on the x-axis and the predicted risk on the y-axis. Note that much of the activity described so far resembles that of Section 4.6 but now we use the validation data.

Using the validation data makes it possible to examine the predictions side by side, for each outcome at the prediction time horizon. Are the outcome positive predictions nicely separated from the outcome negative ones? Or, is there considerable overlap in the predictions between each outcome level, or does one outcome level have a wide distribution while the other one is narrow? These plots are easy to make when the outcome is binary (Section 5.2.1). However, when the outcome is right-censored, with or without competing risks, the censoring issue complicates the calculation. Fortunately we have code that gets around this problem (Sections 5.3.1 and 5.4.1).

Note that our approach above was kept simple, using a single validation dataset. A more rigorous approach would be to use resampling and repeat the above many times.

5.1.2   Calculation of model performance

There are two fundamental metrics that are always calculated for assessing prediction model performance. One is the area under the (time-dependent) receiver operating characteristic (ROC) curve [86, 92, 24]. This is the probability that the patient who experiences the event (until the prediction time horizon) will have a higher predicted probability of the event, relative to the patient who does not experience the event (until the prediction time horizon). Thus, this metric measures the discrimination ability of the model. We will provide code to compute this metric in all of the settings (Sections 5.2.3, 5.3.3, 5.4.3). The other metric we advocate is the Brier score [34] (also known as mean probability score [187]), and derived from it the Index of Prediction Accuracy (IPA) [115]. In short, the Brier score and IPA examine prediction accuracy including calibration, not just discrimination of predicted risks.

When the AUC indicates good performance but the Brier score and IPA indicate bad or even harmful performance, a likely reason is that the model is not well calibrated.

This is explained later, but we also provide code to calculate this in all settings (Section 5.2.2, 5.3.2 and 5.4.2).

5.1.3   Visualization of model performance

The mainstay of model performance visualization is the calibration plot. It shows the expected outcome proportion across the spectrum of predicted probabilities and where those predicted probabilities tend to lie. The x-axis of the calibration plot is the predicted risk of the model. The y-axis of the calibration plot depends on the situation. In uncensored data, the observed frequency of the outcome event is calculated simply by counting (Section 5.2.4). In right-censored data with and without competing risks, the actual risk is estimated using the Kaplan-Meier (Section 5.3.4) and the Aalen-Johansen methods (Section 5.4.4), respectively. Ideally, the calibration curve would follow the 45-degree line so that predicted probabilities always match the observed frequency (estimated actual risk) of the event. This never happens; there will always be some deviation, but the degree of deviation can be very informative.

For example, considering a calibration plot, we may see that at very high predicted risks, the predictions are too high, i.e., the calibration curve is clearly below the 45-degree line. We may also see that at very low predicted risks, the predictions are too low. So at both ends of the spectrum, the predictions are too extreme. Whether such visual findings reflect real calibration problems depends on how many patients in the population have their predicted risk in the area where the curve deviates. Overlaid on the calibration plot is therefore information on where the predictions tend to lie. This is useful for the interpretation of the curve. It is also useful to note whether the discrepancies at the extremes matter in practice. If a predicted probability is a little too high, but the observed is still very high, this miscalibration may not matter because the patient is already at sufficiently high risk. This same issue can occur at very low predictions.

A calibration plot is mostly a graphical tool very much like a histogram or density plot. Hence, any attempt to summarize calibration performance in a single number [13] should always be accompanied by the actual calibration plot. There are two commonly used types of calibration plot: the histogram type and the density type. The histogram type of calibration plot (e.g., Figure 5.7) has some clear limitations: it has an intrinsic "user bias" as it depends crucially on the number of risk groups chosen (see Section 5.2.4); it cannot show two or more models in one graph; and it distorts the x-axis. The density type of calibration plot (e.g., Figure 5.9) depends on a smoothing parameter called the bandwidth, but this is usually chosen by the computer and hence less prone to user bias. So, for the histogram, the choice of the bins is arbitrary, and for the smooth plot, the method of smoothing is arbitrary. As such, either one is vulnerable to modeler manipulation. In our view, the smoothed plot is easier to visualize, so we will more commonly present calibration this way.

Another popular visualization choice is the ROC curve. This curve nicely illustrates the tradeoff between sensitivity and specificity as the threshold is varied across the scale of the predicted probabilities. However, one must be cautious when using this curve or the area under it for decision-making purposes (Section 2.1.7, 9.1). Investigators might want to choose the threshold that leads to the optimal value of sensitivity and specificity. However, this method is inappropriate for determining a clinical threshold because it does not optimize clinical utility [85, 97, 182]. Nevertheless, ROC curves are useful at earlier stages of the modeling process, and we show examples of ROC curves in all three settings (Section 5.2.3, 5.3.3 and 5.4.3).

5.2 Uncensored binary outcome

This setting is characterized by the uncensored outcome: no one is lost to follow-up before the prediction time horizon, and hence, the outcome status (event yes or no) of all test set subjects is known at the prediction time horizon. Recall also from Section 4.1.1 that this setting allows that competing risks happen to some subjects before the time horizon; their event status is zero (no event). In other words, the subjects who experience a competing risk before the prediction time horizon are mixed together with the subjects who are free of all events at the time origin, as both groups have event status zero.

5.2.1 Distribution of the predicted risks

Before analyzing prediction performance it is useful to visualize the distribution of the predicted risks. To do this, the initial step is to use the model to evaluate the predicted risks of the test set subjects. Then, standard tools of basic statistics can be used to summarize and visualize the distribution across the test set, subsets thereof, and also conditional on the outcome at the prediction horizon.

For illustration consider the in vitro fertilization study. Here we obtain the risks of ovarian hyperstimulation syndrome (OHSS) for 102 test set patients by applying a logistic regression model that was trained using the training dataset. The parameter estimates (regression coefficients as odds ratios) of this model are shown in Table 5.1.

We add the predicted risks to the test set and show the first five and the last five subjects (Table 5.2). Even though the subjects were not sorted in any way, Table 5.2 readily shows that the predicted risks vary from very low (subject 1) to very high (subject 102). To get a more complete picture one can, for example, choose a box plot, a density plot, or a histogram. Figure 5.1 illustrates the distribution of predicted risk across all 102 test set subjects. This is a useful graph to see how many subjects actually receive very high and how many very low predicted risks.

Another useful illustration of the predicted risks in the test dataset is to visualize the variation of predicted risks according to the values of single

TABLE 5.1
In vitro fertilization study. Logistic regression results based on the training set.

Variable	Units	OddsRatio	CI.95	p-value
No. antral follicles		1.15	[1.09;1.21]	< 0.01
Cycle length		1.13	[0.94;1.37]	0.201
Age		0.95	[0.85;1.07]	0.402
Smoking status	No	Ref		
	Yes	0.39	[0.16;0.94]	0.036

TABLE 5.2
In vitro fertilization study. Risk predictions of logistic regression model for first 5 and last 5 subjects in test dataset. The first column is a running subject number. The second column (OHSS) contains the outcome (0: no OHSS, 1: OHSS), columns 3-5 the subject characteristics, and the last column shows the risks predicted by the logistic regression model (c.f., Table 5.1).

id	ohss	ant.foll	cyclelen	age	smoking	risk.ohss
1	0	5	28	32	Yes	2.5
2	0	13	30	25	Yes	12.0
3	1	30	32	36	No	72.7
4	0	22	29	37	No	37.2
5	0	25	31	30	No	61.3
98	0	17	28	32	No	25.1
99	0	16	28	32	No	22.7
100	0	26	29	35	No	52.8
101	0	12	28	36	No	12.4
102	1	51	28	32	No	97.1

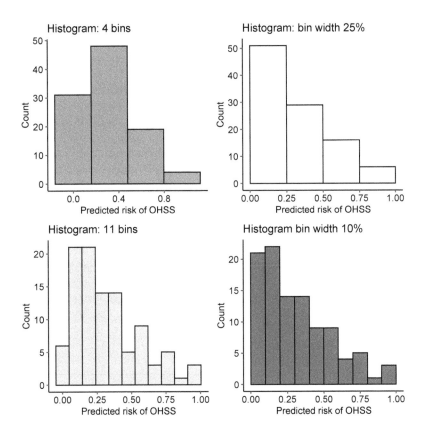

FIGURE 5.1
In vitro fertilization study. Distribution of predicted risks obtained with a logistic regression model (Table 5.1) across test set subjects. All four histograms show the same data.

predictor variables. The purpose of this type of graph is mostly descriptive because the outcome of the test set subjects is not used. It can, however, illustrate the relative importance of a predictor variable for the prediction model. It is also possible to show how the predicted risks vary according to a variable that was not used by the prediction model, but the interpretation would be less obvious. With few predictor variables, one can squeeze multiple similar graphs into one figure. With many predictor variables one can conveniently use a multi-page device such as PDF. To illustrate this concept, Figure 5.2 shows how the predicted risks of the test set subjects of our in vitro fertilization study vary according to the 4 variables that were used by the logistic regression model to create the predictions. It is clearly visible that age and cycle length are less important for the prediction model than the number of antral follicles. For a given value of age, say 32 years, the predicted risks vary between 0 and 100% whereas for any given value of the number of antral follicles the risks do not vary by much. Smoking status seems to be important too, with smokers receiving systematically lower predicted risks than non-smokers.

In the uncensored outcome setting, it is also straightforward to illustrate the distribution of the predicted risks conditional on the outcome. For example, one can show boxplots of the predicted risks for those subjects who at the prediction time horizon have the event and for those who do not. When there are competing risks it will typically be useful to show one boxplot for the predicted risks given to subjects who had a competing risk and one boxplot for the predicted risks given to subjects who were event-free at the prediction time horizon.

Figure 5.3 shows boxplots of predicted risks of ovarian hyperstimulation syndrome conditional on the outcome of test set patients. One should recognize that even though it is tempting to interpret this type of graph immediately as prediction performance it is mainly useful to describe the predicted risks. The following R-code produces the plot.

```
# R-code
fit <- glm(ohss~ant.foll+cyclelen+age+smoking,data=ivftrain,family=
    "binomial")
x <- Score(list(fit),formula=ohss~1,data=ivftest,summary="
    riskQuantiles")
boxplot(x)
abline(v=mean(ivftest$ohss),lty=2)
abline(v=mean(predictRisk(fit,newdata=ivftest)),lty=3)
```

The boxplot clearly shows that most of the patients who actually have the outcome are also receiving higher predicted risks than most of the patients who do not have the outcome. Even though boxplots conditional on the outcome provide a nice way of visualizing the distribution of the predicted risks, one cannot easily translate the graph into a metric for assessing prediction performance. The problem is that a proper interpretation of the boxplots requires that the models are calibrated. The logistic regression model would be

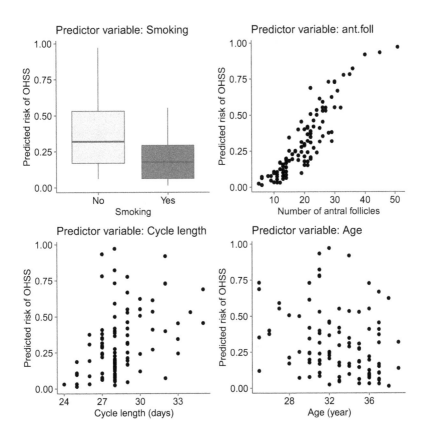

FIGURE 5.2

In vitro fertilization study. Distribution of predicted risks obtained with a logistic regression model (Table 5.1) across test set subjects. All four histograms show the same data.

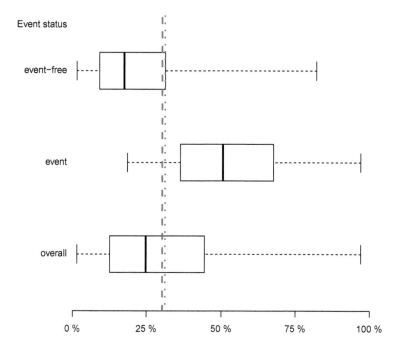

FIGURE 5.3
Boxplots showing predicted risks of OHSS conditional on the outcome of the test set patients. The vertical dashed line is the outcome prevalence in the test set patients and the dotted line is the average of the predicted risks of the test set patients according to the logistic regression model.

perfectly calibrated *in the large* (see Section 2.2.2) if the dashed dotted line and the dashed line were indistinguishable in Figure 5.3.

5.2.2 Brier score

A natural and meaningful way to compare the predicted risk (a number between 0 and 100%) to the outcome (0 if the event did not occur or 1 if the event occurred) is the average distance between them. For a single person, the Brier score is the mean of the squared difference between the subject's predicted risk and his outcome. To calculate the Brier score (in a test set) we first apply the model to obtain predicted risks of all subjects and then compare these to the actual outcomes. The Brier score of the model is the average of the squared differences between the predicted risks and outcomes. Thus, the Brier score is nothing else than the mean squared error of prediction. By taking the square root of the Brier score, we obtain an interpretation as the average distance between the predicted risk and the outcome. Since the Brier score is a population average it does not have a direct interpretation for the single patient, however, the population average Brier score can be used to compare models and to identify the best risk prediction model (in terms of average prediction performance).

> *The interpretation of the Brier score of a model works by comparison with benchmark values and those of rival models.*

The Brier score provides values between zero and one, with a lower value indicating better model performance. There are a few benchmarks that a useful model should outperform. If instead of using a model, one would predict a random probability, one would achieve a Brier score of 33%. If one predicts 50% risk for all subjects, this corresponds to saying "I have no information about your outcome," and one achieves a Brier score of 25%. See Table 5.3 for a summary of these benchmark values. However, in order to evaluate your model you want to compare it to the null model that predicts the test set prevalence of the outcome to all subjects (Figure 5.4). Note that the Brier score appropriately penalizes a procedure that flips a coin or a random number between 0 and 100% relative to predicting 50% for everyone. The former predictions are worse because they would push someone inappropriately toward a decision with extreme (but random) predictions. Such predictions are harmful and useless. Always predicting 50% is not harmful but is useless.

To illustrate the computation of the Brier score in the case of uncensored binary outcome data we consider a logistic regression model fitted to the training dataset of the in vitro fertilization study. The model predicts the risk of ovarian hyperstimulation syndrome (*ohss*) based on the number of antral follicles (*ant.foll*), cycle length, age and smoking status. Table 5.1 shows the odds ratios with confidence limits.

A higher number of antral follicles is associated with a higher risk and both

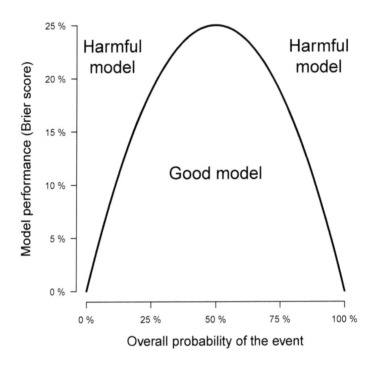

FIGURE 5.4
Benchmark values for the Brier score. The solid line is the Brier score of the null model, which predicts the overall probability of the event to all subjects. The null model ignores the predictor variables. A good model uses the predictor variables and outperforms the null model.

TABLE 5.3
Benchmark values for the AUC (concordance index) and Brier score at any fixed prediction time horizon t. See Figure 5.4 for an illustration of the most important benchmark: the null model which ignores the predictor variables.

Benchmark prediction	AUC	Brier score	Interpretation
50% always	50%	25%	useless or harmful
Overall event probability always	50%	see Figure 5.4	useless
Coin toss	50%	50%	harmful
Uniform [0,1]	50%	33%	harmful

higher age and smoking are associated with lower risk. In order to evaluate
how well the model can predict ovarian hyperstimulation syndrome we apply
it to 6 selected subjects of the test dataset (Table 5.4). The table shows
outcome (*ohss*) and predicted risks (*Risk*) for these 6 subjects. The predicted
risk is obtained with the logistic regression model shown in Table 5.1 using
the covariate data (*ant.foll, age, Smoking*). The last column (*Brier residual*)
shows the subject-specific squared differences between the outcome and the
predicted risk. The subjects without the event (OHSS) have a small residual
if their predicted risk is low, and the subjects with the event (OHSS) have a
small residual if their predicted risk is high.

TABLE 5.4
In vitro fertilization study. Shown are Brier score residuals (*ohss −*
predicted risk)^2 for 6 patients of the test dataset. The predicted risks are obtained with the logistic regression model shown in Table 5.1. The Brier score
of the model is the average of the Brier score residuals across all patients in
the test dataset.

ID	ant.foll	age	smoking	ohss	Predicted risk	Brier residual
15	21	30	Yes	1	0.241	0.576
31	19	34	No	0	0.312	0.097
52	27	36	No	0	0.550	0.302
69	22	34	No	0	0.347	0.120
71	24	29	No	1	0.500	0.250
87	9	33	Yes	0	0.046	0.002

In independent test data (uncensored), the standard error of the Brier
score is calculated as the square root of the standard deviation of the
squared residuals. Based on this we implement Wald-type confidence
intervals and tests.

The Brier score of the logistic regression model (Table 5.1) across all test
set patients is computed as follows:

```
# R-code
fit <- glm(ohss~ant.foll+cyclelen+age+smoking,data=ivftrain,family=
    "binomial")
Score(list("My model"=fit),formula=ohss~1,data=ivftest,metrics="
    brier",summary="ipa")
```

Metric Brier:

Results by model:

```
model Brier lower upper   IPA
1: Null model   21.2  17.6  24.7  0.0
2:   My model   14.0  10.5  17.4 34.1
```

Results of model comparisons:

```
       model  reference delta.Brier lower upper              p
1: My model Null model        -7.2 -10.6  -3.8 0.00003019228
```

NOTE: Values are multiplied by 100 and given in %
NOTE: The lower Brier the better, the higher IPA the better.

The prevalence of ovarian hyperstimulation syndrome in the test set of our in vitro fertilization study is 30.4% and hence the benchmark Brier score of the null model is 21.2% (see Figure 5.4). The Brier score of the logistic regression model is much lower than the null model's score, indicating that the model based on these covariates has some ability for predicting the risk of ovarian hyperstimulation syndrome. A formal test shows that the Brier score of the logistic regression model is significantly lower by 7.2% (CI-95%: [3.8%; 10.6%]) than that of the null model ($p < 0.0001$).

5.2.3   AUC

A concordance statistic quantifies the ability of the model to correctly order patients by their predicted risks. In the binary setting, this discrimination statistic is also known as the area under the ROC curve (AUC) or c-statistic, and the interpretation is as follows. For a randomly chosen pair of subjects, where one subject has the event and one has not, the concordance index is the probability that the model assigns the higher risk to the subject who has the event.

Being a rank statistic, the AUC is blind to miscalibration of the predicted risks. Hence, it cannot stand alone to assess models with respect to predictive accuracy.

To compute the AUC for your model, the computer first constructs all possible pairs of subjects in the test dataset. The computer next excludes pairs where both subjects have the same outcome. Now the predicted risks are used to group the remaining pairs into concordant, discordant and tied predictions. A concordant pair means that the patient who has the event had the higher predicted risk. A discordant pair means that the patient who has the event has the lower predicted risk. Tied pairs indicate that both patients have exactly the same predicted risks. Finally, the AUC is calculated as the number of concordant pairs plus half of the tied pairs divided by the total number of pairs. For further illustration see Table 5.5.

The AUC of the logistic regression model (Table 5.1) in the test dataset is obtained with the following R-code.

```
# R-code
fit <- glm(ohss~ant.foll+cyclelen+age+smoking,data=ivftrain,family=
    "binomial")
Score(list("My model"=fit),formula=ohss~1,data=ivftest,metrics="auc
    ")
```

Metric AUC:

Results by model:

```
       model  AUC lower upper
1: My model 86.5  79.5  93.5
```

NOTE: Values are multiplied by 100 and given in %.
NOTE: The higher AUC the better.

Now that you know the concordance index (AUC) of your model, what does it mean? A value of 100% means that all pairs of subjects were correctly ranked. In practice, this rarely happens. A value of 50% means that the prediction model is no good; it does not discriminate. The reason is that we can obtain this value, AUC = 50%, by flipping a coin or by predicting the same risk for every subject (all pairs are tied). This lower benchmark value 50% is also obtained by an artificial model which predicts a random number between 0% and 100%. Thus, a model with discrimination ability equal to 50% is useless or even harmful. However, note that the AUC cannot tell the difference between a useless and a harmful model.

Other than needing to be larger than 50%, there are no general rules for how large the discrimination of the model has to be – this depends on how heterogeneous the population is with respect to the risk of the event. However, it is sometimes claimed that the AUC above 65% is moderate and above 75% is good, and so on. We do not support this claim because the absolute value of the AUC depends on the case-mix and cannot be compared across different fields of application(Section 2.2.6).

It is important to recognize that these rules have no basis and are potentially meaningless (Figure 5.5). The reason is that the value of the AUC depends on things other than the model: the homogeneity of the population, which is affected by inclusion criteria, and the availability and distribution of the predictor variables.

In a homogeneous population, even the perfect model can have low discrimination ability (AUC). In a heterogeneous population, even a bad model can have a high AUC.

This also means that AUC is generally not comparable between settings. Thus, instead of fixed thresholds for defining a "good" AUC, the best use of

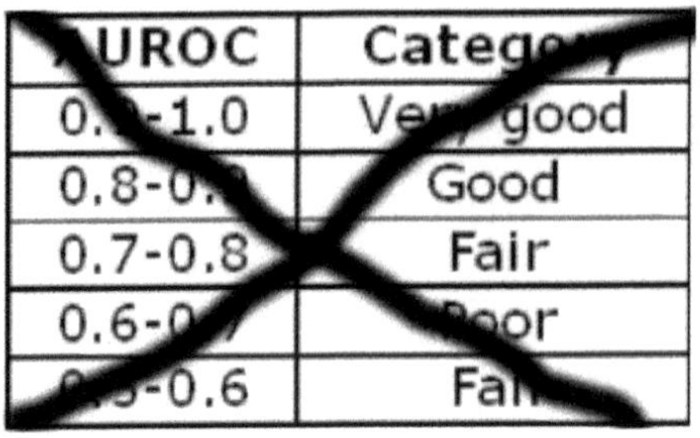

UROC	Category
0.~~~-1.0	Ve~~ good
0.8-0.~	Good
0.7-0.8	Fair
0.6-0~	~~or
~~-0.6	Fa~~

FIGURE 5.5
Interpretation of the AUC: fixed thresholds are not useful to interpret the
AUC (or any other measure of performance), see Section 2.2.6. Instead, a good
model outperforms the benchmark values (Table 5.3) and the rival models
(Chapter 6).

a concordance index is to compare the model with rival model(s) in the same
data that were not used to build a model (Chapter 6).

Table 5.5 illustrates the calculation of the AUC based on pairs of subjects of the test dataset. The logistic regression model scores an AUC value
of 85.6% (CI-95%: [78.2%;92.9%]). Figure 5.6 shows the corresponding ROC
curve. Each point on the ROC curve for a risk prediction model corresponds to
a value p between 0% and 100%. For example, at the threshold $p = 21.6\%$ the
estimates of the sensitivity and specificity are 90.3% and 40.8%, respectively.
The ROC curve (Figure 5.6) can be obtained with the following code:

```
# R-code
fit <- glm(ohss~ant.foll+smoking+age,data=ivftrain,family=binomial)
x <- Score(list("My-model"=fit), data=ivftest, formula=ohss~1,
        plots="ROC")
plotROC(x)
```

It is generally not recommended to estimate an optimal threshold based
on an ROC curve. One problem is that the ROC curve does not incorporate
the prevalence/utility of the medical condition [97]. Another problem is that
a patient with a predicted risk of 0.1% would receive the same answer as a patient with a predicted risk of 18.0% when the threshold 18.1% is implemented.
Finally, a more technical problem is that estimates of thresholds tend to be
highly variable even in large sample sizes (see also Sections 2.1.7 and 9.1).

5.2.4   Calibration curves

A model is well-calibrated (in the large) if 17% of the subjects have the event
when the predicted risk for all of them is 17%. The value 17% is just an
example. This should hold for all values that the predicted risk can take,

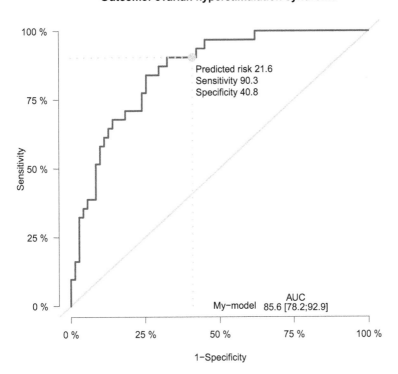

FIGURE 5.6
In vitro fertilization study. ROC curve for a logistic regression model that uses the number of antral follicles, age, and smoking status to predict the risk of ovarian hyperstimulation syndrome. The model was fitted in the training dataset and the ROC curve was calculated in the test dataset. In most cases, it is not useful to base the decision on a threshold value, such as 21.6% risk, solely on the ROC curve (c.f., Chapter 9.1).

TABLE 5.5
The 6 subjects of Table 5.4 are used to illustrate the calculation of the AUC.
In Table 5.4 there are two subjects with ovarian hyperstimulation syndrome
(OHSS). Their predicted risks are shown in the first column and concordance
of the pair (third column) is obtained by comparing with the predicted risk
of each of the four subjects without OHSS shown in the second column. The
AUC is the average of the concordance column across all pairs in the test
dataset where one subject has OHSS and the other does not.

Subjects with OHSS	Subjects without OHSS	Concordance
24.1	31.2	0
24.1	55.0	0
24.1	34.7	0
24.1	4.6	0
50.0	31.2	1
50.0	55.0	0
50.0	34.7	1
50.0	4.6	1

i.e., all values between 0% and 100%. The calibration curve is defined over
the range of values that the model is possibly predicting. For any such value
the calibration is the observed event frequency among patients that have a
predicted risk equal or at least close to that value. There are many different
ways to define "close," and a popular method is to simply categorize the
predicted risks according to deciles [123]. This yields the histogram type of the
calibration plot. Figure 5.7 shows a calibration diagram based on 10 groups of
the predicted risks that are obtained using deciles. The model is well-calibrated
(in the small) if the light gray bars are as high as the dark gray bars.

```
# R-code
fit <- glm(ohss~ant.foll+smoking+age,data=ivftrain,family=binomial)
x <- Score(list("My-model"=fit), data=ivftest, formula=ohss~1,
        plots="calibration")
plotCalibration(x,bars=1,q=10)
```

In Figure 5.7 we see some deviations from perfect calibration, in particular,
in the lower end of the predicted risks. This may indicate that the model is
not nicely calibrated. However, two readers of the same graph may come to
different conclusions regarding how well the model is calibrated. It is therefore
useful to "calibrate the eye." A constructive way to do so was proposed by
Blanche et al. (2019) [25]. The idea is to computer simulate data like the
real data under the assumption that the model is perfectly calibrated. If it
is possible to find the calibration plot corresponding to the real data (where
calibration is unknown) which is hidden in a sequence of calibration plots

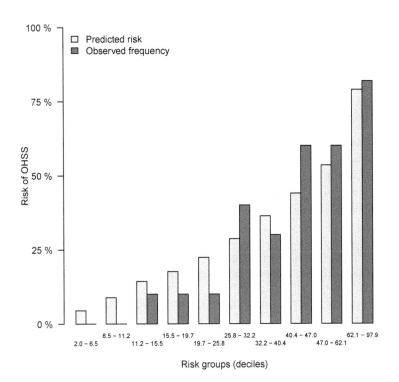

FIGURE 5.7

In vitro fertilization study. Calibration plot (histogram type) for the logistic regression model fitted to the training dataset. The model's risk predictions for the patients in the test dataset are grouped into 10 equally large groups. The values below the x-axis show the thresholds. Within each group the observed frequency is the relative frequency of patients in the test dataset with the outcome (OHSS).

corresponding to simulated data (where calibration is perfect), then the model is miscalibrated.

Another problem is that the histogram type of calibration plot is quite sensitive to the number of groups, as is the corresponding Hosmer-Lemeshow test (Section 9.5). This is illustrated in Figure 5.8 which shows the calibration of the same model as Figure 5.7 but now with 3 groups of the predicted risk obtained with tertiles instead of 10 groups. Now, at least in the medium-risk group the model appears calibrated. But, we are by no means proposing to change the number of groups until the graph looks suitably nice. In order to avoid biased conclusions, the choice of the number of groups should be prespecified or based on some formula as is commonly used to define the number of bars of a histogram.

```
# R-code
plotCalibration(x,bars=1,q=3)
```

As an alternative to the histogram type, one can use the density type of calibration plot. The density type of calibration curve shown in Figure 5.9 is the graph where you have the range of predicted risks on the x-axis and the running average of the corresponding 0-1 outcome values on the y-axis.

```
# R-code
layout(matrix(c(1,2),nrow=2),height=c(.7,0.3))
plotCalibration(x)
boxplot(x$Calibration$plotframe$risk,horizontal=TRUE,
    main="",xlab="",axes=FALSE,ylim=c(0,1))
```

To compute the curve, the computer orders the predicted risks and then defines a window of values around points on the x-axis to be included in the calculation of the observed frequency. However, the density type of the calibration curve is sensitive to the width of the window [77]. Also, when interpreting a local deviation from the diagonal, one needs to consider the number of subjects in that region of the predicted risk.

The calibration curve is attractive because it is a nice graphical representation between the predicted risks and actual outcome. It is user-friendly to interpret because the eye simply judges the gap between the calibration curve and the 45-degree line of the plot. For example, Figure 5.9 indicates an overestimation of the predicted risks in the interval 75%-100%. Here the calibration line is below the diagonal, and hence, the observed event frequency is lower than the predicted risks. Unfortunately, there are three important limitations of the calibration curve. First, it does not quantify the miscalibration of the model as a single number. Second, deviations of the curve from the 45-degree line are more important in regions where many subjects have their predicted risk. Unfortunately the eyeball cannot easily do this weighting. Third, there are numerous ways of calculating the running average and the choice of method typically impacts the visual nature of the curve.

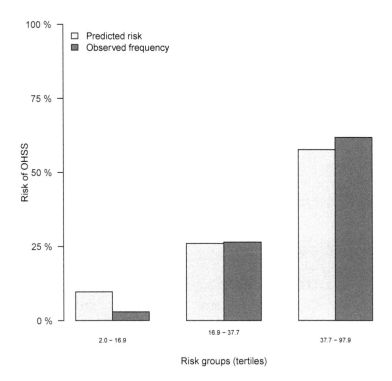

FIGURE 5.8
In vitro fertilization study. Calibration plot (histogram type) for the logistic
regression model fitted to the training dataset. The model's risk predictions
for the patients in the test dataset are grouped into 3 equally large groups. The
values below the x-axis show the thresholds. Within each group the observed
frequency is the relative frequency of patients in the test dataset with the
outcome (OHSS).

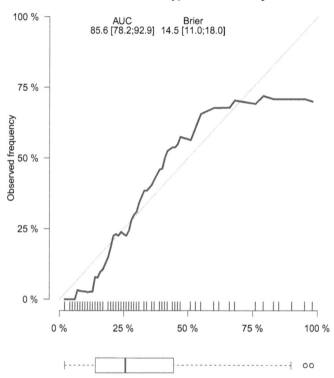

FIGURE 5.9
In vitro fertilization study. Calibration plot (density type) for the logistic regression model fitted to the training dataset. The model's risk predictions for the patients in the test dataset are ordered from low to high. A fixed bandwidth defines how many test dataset patients are nearest neighbors to any given value p on the x-axis. The observed frequency at the value p is the relative frequency of test dataset patients with the outcome (OHSS) in the neighborhood around the value p. The rug plot at the bottom of the diagram and the boxplot below show the distribution of the predicted risks.

5.3 Right-censored time-to-event outcome (without competing risks)

We now consider the situation where the outcome is a right-censored time-to-event variable and the predicted risk is an estimate of the probability that the event occurs until a fixed prediction time horizon. In this section we consider the special case without competing risks. For example, the event of interest could be "death due to any cause" or a combined endpoint such as "relapse or death." Without competing risks the predicted risk is complementary to the predicted survival probability, so from a model which predicts survival chances (until a fixed prediction time horizon) we extract the corresponding predicted risks by subtracting the predicted survival probability from 100%.

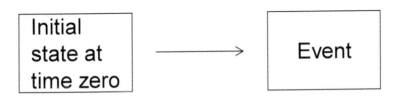

FIGURE 5.10
Two-state model for survival analysis without competing risks. All subjects will experience the event, sooner or later. Censoring means that for some subjects the follow-up time is not long enough to observe the event time.

Something else to note is that, for any fixed prediction time horizon, this setting closely resembles that of the binary setting. The outcome is 1 if the event occurs at some point between the time origin and the prediction horizon, and the outcome is 0 if the subject reaches the horizon without the event. What distinguishes this setting from the binary one is censoring, which is the presence of subjects who have not experienced the event but have not been followed until the horizon. For these subjects, the event status at the prediction time horizon is unknown (see Section 4.6.2). Simply removing subjects with unknown status is not acceptable as it introduces bias.

Generally, with right-censored data, the objective remains the same as it would be if the data were uncensored. That is, we define the prediction performance parameters (AUC, Brier score, IPA) in the ideal setting where no subject is lost to follow-up before the prediction time horizon. The challenge is to estimate the parameters based on the right-censored data. To do this we use a specific statistical weighting technique called *inverse probability of censoring weighting* [82, 74, 24]. In order to avoid division with zero, this technique makes the assumption that the probability of not being censored at the time horizon is strictly positive. In a theoretical sense, this positivity assumption is needed for all combinations of the predictor variables that a single subject can possibly have. In Section 5.6 we explain how to check this assumption.

5.3.1   Distribution of the predicted risks

As in the uncensored case (Section 5.2.1), it is illustrative to visualize the distribution of the predicted risks conditional on the outcome at the prediction time horizon. It is difficult to display biomarker or predicted values with respect to the outcome when the outcome involves censored data. While boxplots of the events and nonevents would be nice to visualize, the censored observations do not naturally belong in either boxplot nor can they be excluded without bias. To adapt the boxplot displays to accommodate censored data, including when competing risks are present, we estimate quantiles of the predicted risks conditional on the outcome status at a fixed time horizon. Particularly, we use a so-called *inverse of the probability of censoring weighted* estimator. We illustrate the R-code with examples to produce the desired boxplots. These displays help illustrate how the specific biomarker values vary with the survival-type outcome. Our R-code should be useful to researchers who wish to illustrate how their novel biomarkers or risk prediction model helps discriminate among time-to-event outcomes [113].

To illustrate this, we fit a Cox regression model to the training set of the oral cancer data adjusted for *age*, *tumorthickness* and *grade*. The regression coefficients (hazard ratios) of the Cox regression model are shown in Table 5.6.

TABLE 5.6
Oral cancer study. Cox regression results based on the training set.

Variable	Units	HazardRatio	CI.95	p-value
age	years	1.03	[1.02;1.04]	< 0.001
tumorthickness	mm	1.49	[1.36;1.63]	< 0.001
grade	Well	Ref		
	Moderate	1.34	[1.04;1.73]	0.0239
	Poor	1.37	[0.98;1.92]	0.0665

Figure 5.11 illustrates the boxplots conditional on the outcome where the 10-year predicted risks of mortality are obtained by applying the Cox regression model to the test set patients. We see that most patients (more than 50%) who died within 10 years received a higher predicted risk than the average and most patients who survived 10 years received a lower predicted risk than the average.

```
# R-code
fit <- coxph(Surv(survtime,survstatus)~age+tumorthickness+grade,
    data=octrain,x=1)
x <- Score(list("My-model"=fit),
    formula=Surv(survtime,survstatus)~1, data=octest,
    times=120, summary=c("riskQuantiles"), null.model=0)
boxplot(x,event.labels=c("Overall","Dead","Alive"),outcome.label="
    10-year\nmortality")
```

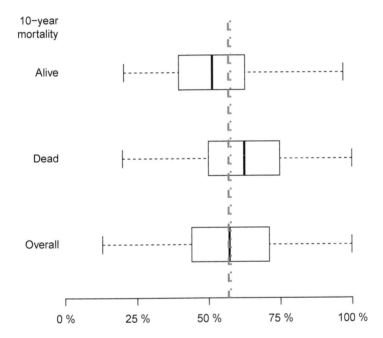

FIGURE 5.11
Oral cancer study. Boxplots showing the predicted 10-year mortality risks
of a Cox regression model conditional on the 10-year outcome. The boxplot
labeled "Overall" shows observed quantiles of 10-year mortality risks in all
test set patients. The boxplots labeled "Alive" and "Dead" are estimated
using the inverse probability of censoring weighting. The vertical dashed line
is the Kaplan-Meier estimate in the test dataset and the vertical dotted line
is the average of the Cox model's risk predictions in the test dataset.

5.3.2   Brier score with censored data

The inverse probability of censoring weighted estimate of the average Brier score is obtained as follows. The test set data are divided into three groups with respect to a given prediction time horizon:

- Group *event*: contains all subjects who experience the event before the prediction time horizon.

- Group *event-free*: contains all subjects who were followed without the event until the prediction time horizon.

- Group *censored*: contains all subjects that are lost to follow-up before the prediction time horizon.

To obtain the estimate of the average Brier score we calculate the squared distance for the subjects in the groups where the event status at the prediction time horizon is known (groups *event* and *event-free*). Instead of a simple average, we calculate a weighted average to account for differences in lengths of follow-up. The weights attached to subjects belonging to the *event* group are evaluated at their individual event times, whereas the weights in the *event-free* group get weights that are evaluated at the prediction time horizon. Note that it does not matter whether any of the subjects who were observed event-free until the prediction time horizon are later observed to experience the event (after the prediction time horizon); outcomes after the prediction time horizon are ignored. Subjects in the *censored* group are not directly used in the weighted average. However, they enter indirectly through the weights assigned to other subjects. The weight given to uncensored subjects is higher the more subjects were lost to follow-up (*censored*) earlier in time. This is to account for the fact that those in the *censored* group could possibly have experienced the event by the prediction time horizon, just this is not observed [79]. It is possible and sometimes useful to let the weights also depend on subject-specific baseline characteristics. However, typically the weights are obtained with the Kaplan-Meier method for the censored times [82] in which case, the weights do not depend on the baseline characteristics. Unfortunately, this can lead to bias in cases where the length of the follow-up period depends on the baseline covariates, and in this instance, more sophisticated modeling may be necessary. For example, a Cox regression model can be fitted to the censoring times to obtain the weights [74].

We illustrate the calculation of the weighted Brier score using a Cox regression model fitted in the training set of the oral cancer data. Based on the model shown in Table 5.6, we predict the 10-year all-cause mortality risk in the test set of the oral cancer study. Table 5.7 shows the predicted 10-year mortality risks of 6 selected patients. The *time* is given in months, and the prediction time horizon is set at 120 months (10 years). The Brier score residuals are calculated as the square of 1 minus the predicted risks for subjects with an event time before the prediction time horizon and as the square of

0 minus the predicted risks for subjects with an event time larger than the prediction time horizon (even if no event has not yet happened). The column *IPCW* shows the inverse probability of censoring weights according to the Kaplan-Meier estimate of the censoring survival function in the test set (Figure 5.12, right panel).

```
# R-code
# Kaplan-Meier:
F <- prodlim(Hist(survtime,survstatus)~1,data=octest)
plot(F)
# reverse Kaplan-Meier
G <- prodlim(Hist(survtime,survstatus)~1,data=octest,reverse=1)
plot(G)
```

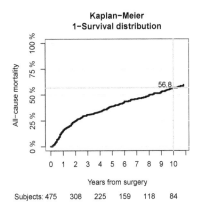 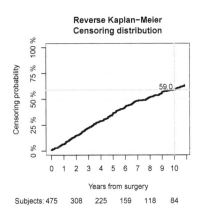

FIGURE 5.12

Oral cancer study. Kaplan-Meier and reverse Kaplan-Meier calculated in the test set patients. The gray lines in the left panel indicate the predicted risk of the null model at the 10-year prediction time horizon. The gray lines in the right panel show that 59.0% of the patients were lost to follow-up alive within 10 years from surgery.

The second patient in Table 5.7 was alive after 33 months and then lost to follow-up. Hence the 10-year outcome for this patient is unknown, and the IPCW weight is zero. The same is true for the fifth patient. The first patient died after 11 months, and the Cox model's predicted 10-year mortality risk (based on *age*, *tumorthickness* and *grade*) is 90.0%. The weight attached to this patient is obtained as one divided by the probability of end of follow up (AKA the inverse probability of censoring) evaluated at 11 months (Figure 5.12, right panel). The weights of the 3rd and 4th patients in Table 5.7, who are also in group *event*, are obtained similarly with the reverse Kaplan-Meier evaluated at 50 and 96 months, respectively. The last patient in Table 5.7 is in group *event-free*, but the survival status at the prediction time horizon is known: *alive*. The residual is weighted with one divided by the inverse probability of censoring evaluated at 120 months. According to Figure 5.12 (right panel) the cumulative probability of censoring (end of follow-up probability) at 10 years is 59.0%. The inverse probability of censoring is therefore 100.0% – 59.0% = 41.0% and the weight shown in Table 5.7 given to the sixth subject is $1/0.41 = 2.44$.

TABLE 5.7
Oral cancer study. Calculation of weighted Brier score residuals. Shown are outcome data (*time, status*) and 10-year mortality risk predictions of 6 patients of the test dataset. See discussion of the contributions to the Brier score at the prediction time in the text.

Time	Status	Outcome 10-yrs	Predicted 10-yrs risk	Brier residuals	IPCW	Weighted residuals
11	1	1	0.90	0.01	1.07	0.01
33	0	unknown	0.56	unknown	0.00	0.00
50	1	1	0.73	0.08	1.41	0.11
96	1	1	0.54	0.21	2.06	0.43
108	0	unknown	0.53	unknown	0.00	0.00
136	0	0	0.45	0.21	2.44	0.50

The weighted average Brier score across all test set patients is computed as 23.2% (CI-95% [20.2%;26.1%]). The value can be interpreted as the average distance between the predicted 10-year risks and the actual binary outcome at the 10-year horizon (alive or dead).

The theory in [74] tells us that the estimate of the Brier score at the prediction time horizon is unbiased in sufficiently large samples and when the model used to derive the weights is correctly specified.

The interpretation of whether this indicates a good prediction performance of the Cox regression model is done relative to the benchmarks for the Brier score. All data-independent benchmarks for the Brier score remain the same as in the binary setting (Table 5.3). But, with censored data, the null model which predicts the same event risk to all subjects is now obtained as the complement of the Kaplan-Meier estimate of survival evaluated at the prediction time horizon [82, 78]. It is possible to calculate two different null models; one in the training dataset and one in the test dataset. We here chose to apply the Kaplan-Meier method in the test dataset to obtain the null model. That is, the 10-year mortality risk that the null model assigns to all test set subjects is 56.8%, see Figure 5.12 (left panel). The corresponding benchmark for the Brier score is 24.5%. The Brier score of our Cox regression model is lower, indicating that the Cox regression model using the three variables (*age, tumorthickness, grade*) is predictive, but its confidence limits include this benchmark value. It may be of interest to perform a formal test of the null hypothesis that the Brier score of the Cox model is equal to the Brier score of the null model at a fixed prediction time horizon. Such a test can be based on the standard error formula of Blanche et al. [27]. This test shows that the Brier score of the Cox model is not significantly lower than that of the null model ($p > 5\%$) at the 10-year prediction time horizon. Hence, within the limitations of the available data, we cannot conclude that this particular Cox regression model is more useful than not using the covariates and predicting the same predicted risk value to all new patients.

```
# R-code
fit <- coxph(Surv(survtime,survstatus)~age+tumorthickness+grade,
    data=octrain,x=1)
x <- Score(list("Cox"=fit),
        data=octest,
        formula=Surv(survtime,survstatus)~1,
        times=120,
        metrics="brier")
x
```

Metric Brier:

Results by model:

```
          model times Brier lower upper
1: Null model    120  24.5  22.4  26.7
2:          Cox   120  23.2  20.2  26.1
```

Results of model comparisons:

```
   times model   reference delta.Brier lower upper         p
1:   120  Cox Null model        -1.4  -3.6   0.9 0.2368486
```

NOTE: Values are multiplied by 100 and given in %.
NOTE: The lower Brier the better.

5.3.3   Time-dependent AUC for censored data

The inverse probability of censoring weighted estimate of the area under the time-dependent ROC curve (AUC) is computed as follows for any fixed prediction time horizon. The objective remains to calculate the relative frequency of concordant pairs among all pairs in the test data. First, all possible pairs of subjects are formed. Then weights are used to deal with the censoring issue: subjects who have the event are weighted with the probability of being followed until their event time and subjects who are event-free until the prediction time horizon are weighted with the probability of being followed until the prediction horizon. Thus, such a pair is weighted with the product of the two subjects' weights. This may not be totally intuitive but the sum of weighted concordant pairs divided by the sum of weighted pairs is an unbiased estimate of the time-dependent AUC [24].

The theory in [24] tells us that the estimate of the AUC at the prediction time horizon is unbiased in sufficiently large samples and when the model used to derive the weights is correctly specified.

For the purpose of illustration, we calculate the 10-year AUC for the Cox regression model that has been trained in the training set of the oral cancer data. The regression coefficients of the Cox regression model are shown in Table 5.6. As for the illustration of the weighted Brier score, we estimate the inverse probability of censoring weights with the Kaplan-Meier estimate (Figure 5.12 right panel). This means that we implicitly rely on the fact that the length of the potential follow-up time does not depend on the patients' baseline characteristics or on other unobserved confounders. The weighted estimate of the 10-year AUC is obtained as follows.

```
# R-code
fit <- coxph(Surv(survtime,survstatus)~age+tumorthickness+grade,
    data=octrain,x=1)
x <- Score(list("Cox regression"=fit),
      data=octest,
      formula=Surv(survtime,survstatus)~1,
      times=120,
      metrics="auc")
x
```

```
Metric AUC:

Results by model:

          model times  AUC lower upper
1: Cox regression   120 65.3  58.3  72.4

NOTE: Values are multiplied by 100 and given in %.
NOTE: The higher AUC the better.
```

The interpretation of the value of the AUC is as follows: the probability that the Cox regression model assigns a higher predicted 10-year mortality risk to a randomly selected patient who dies within 10 years compared to a randomly selected patient who survives the 10-year period is 65.3% [58.3%;72.4%]. The corresponding ROC curve is shown in Figure 5.13.

```
# R-code
fit <- coxph(Surv(survtime,survstatus)~age+tumorthickness+grade,
    data=octrain,x=1L)
x <- Score(list("Cox"=fit),data=octest,
        formula=Surv(survtime,survstatus)~1,
        times=120,plots="ROC")
plotROC(x, plot.main="Outcome: 10-year all-cause mortality",auc=1)
```

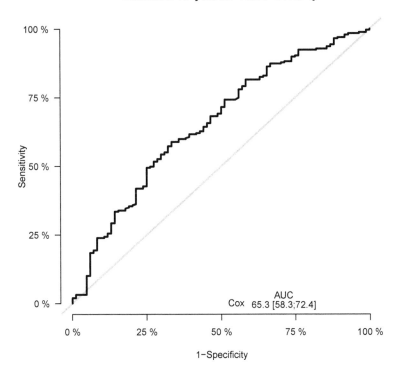

FIGURE 5.13

Oral cancer study. ROC curve for a Cox regression model fitted to the training set. The model uses patient's age, tumor thickness, and grade to predict the 10-year risk of all-cause mortality in the test set of the oral cancer data. The values of the curve and its area are estimated using inverse probability of censoring weights.

5.3.4 Calibration curve for censored data

Visualization and interpretation of the calibration curve remain the same as in
the binary setting. The only difference is the way the average outcome on the
vertical axis is calculated. A popular way to do this is to use the Kaplan-Meier
technique. Another method, which leads to similar results in certain cases
(when censoring is not affected by predictor variables), is the so-called pseudo-
value approach [77]. Figure 5.14 shows the calibration curve for the predicted
10-year risks of the test set patients of the oral cancer data. The predictions
are obtained with the Cox regression model fitted to the training set of the oral
cancer data (Table 5.6). As in the binary uncensored case, the calibration curve
is obtained as a running average across the predicted risks. A disadvantage
with the pseudo-value approach is that the estimation method requires that
the censoring is independent of the covariates. When calculating the running
average across the predicted risks, the option /cens.method="local"/is used
in the R-code below. Instead of using pseudo-values, in this case the Kaplan-
Meier method is applied locally using those test set patients who have received
a predicted risk close to the current value on the x-axis. The value on the y-axis
is thus the Kaplan-Meier estimate of the event probability at the prediction
time horizon. The number of test set subjects that are close at a certain value
can be controlled by the *bandwidth* argument of the function *plotCalibration*.
The default is to let the computer find an optimal value [77].

```
# R-code
fit <- coxph(Surv(survtime,survstatus)~age+tumorthickness+grade,
    data=octrain,x=1L)
x <- Score(list("Cox"=fit), data=octest,
        formula=Surv(survtime,survstatus)~1,
        times=120, plots="calibration")
layout(matrix(c(1,2),nrow=2),height=c(.7,0.3))
plotCalibration(x, pseudo=0, rug=1, cens.method="local",
    plot.main="Outcome: 10 year all-cause mortality")
boxplot(x$Calibration$plotframe$risk,horizontal=TRUE,
    main="",xlab="",axes=FALSE,ylim=c(0,1))
```

We shall also illustrate that calibration plots indicate the spread of predicted risks. Panel A of Figure 5.15 shows that without predictor variables the
spread is zero; the predicted risk based on the training set Kaplan-Meier estimate is 59.1% (Figure 4.1). It also shows that the average 10-year mortality is
slightly higher in the training set compared to the test set, i.e., the black dot
is below the diagonal. Panel B shows the calibration results for a simple Cox
regression model which includes a discrete predictor variable (tumor grade) –
with discrete predictor variables, there is no calibration curve: only calibration
points. We see that the predicted risk based on a Cox regression model fitted
to the training set of the oral cancer data is not perfectly calibrated according
to the estimate of calibration in the test set. In particular, there is some deviation from the diagonal in the group of patients with a "Poor" grade where

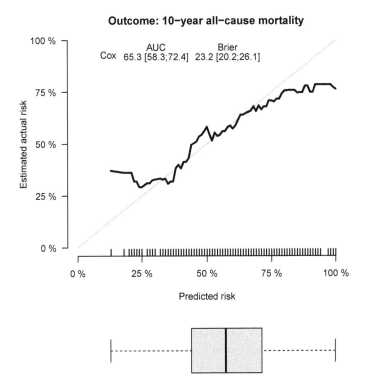

FIGURE 5.14
Oral cancer study. Calibration curve for the Cox regression model fitted to the training set. The model uses patient's age, tumor thickness, and grade to predict the 10-year risk of all-cause mortality in the test set. The rug plot at the bottom and the boxplot below show the distribution of the predicted 10-year mortality risks.

the prediction model predicts a too high value relative to the test set patients in the "Poor" grade group. Panel C shows that a Cox regression model with a single continuous covariate, here patient age, can scatter the predicted risks of individuals quite a bit more. The spread is even larger when we add further variables as in Panel D of Figure 5.15.

5.4   Competing risks

With competing risks, the risk of the event of interest depends on both the hazard rate of the event of interest and the hazard rate of the competing risks. The null model is obtained with the Aalen-Johansen estimator either in the training set (Figure 4.2) or in the validation set (Figure 5.16, Panel A).

In order to estimate the absolute risk of the event of interest conditional on patient characteristics, one option is to combine cause-specific Cox regression models, one for the event of interest and one for the competing risks (see Section 4.1.3) [17, 135]. Based on the same models, one could, in principle, also predict the absolute risk of the competing risk; however, this does not always have an intuitive interpretation when the event of interest is not fatal (as indicated by the dotted arrow in Figure 5.17). For example, when the event of interest is disease progression, and the competing risk is death without disease progression, then it may not be so interesting to know the risk of death without progression, but interesting to know the unconditional risk of death until the prediction time horizon. Another possibility is to predict the risk of the event *progression or death* for which there are no competing risks, and the methods in Section 5.3 apply. In this section, we discuss the prediction performance metrics in the situation with competing risks.

5.4.1   Distribution of the predicted risks

As in the case without competing risks (Section 5.3.1), it is illustrative to visualize the distribution of the predicted risks conditional on the outcome status at the prediction time horizon. With competing risks, there is at least one additional outcome status value at the prediction time horizon: the subject may have experienced a competing risk between time zero and the prediction time horizon. Such a person should receive a relatively lower predicted risk of the event of interest compared to a person who experiences the event of interest before the prediction time horizon. However, with right-censored data, the outcome is not known for all subjects, and the quantiles of the distribution of predicted risks need to be estimated. We have implemented inverse probability of censoring weights to estimate the quantiles of the predicted risks of a model [113].

To illustrate this in the active surveillance prostate cancer study, we fit

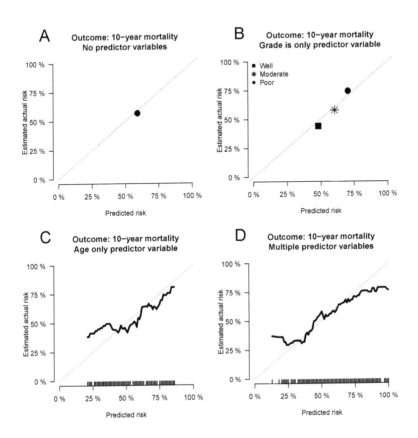

FIGURE 5.15

Oral cancer study. Calibration curves for 4 different models. Panel A shows the predicted risk without any predictor variables obtained with the Kaplan-Meier in the training set (x-axis) vs. the Kaplan-Meier in the test set (y-axis). Panel B shows a Cox regression model which uses only the tumor grade as the only predictor variable. Panel C shows a Cox regression model which uses only patients' age as the only predictor variable. Panel C shows a Cox regression model which uses patients' age, tumor thickness, and grade to predict the 10-year risk of all-cause mortality in the test set of the oral cancer data.

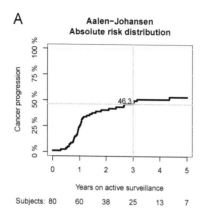
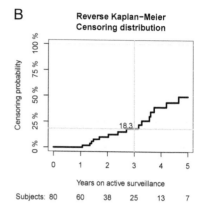

FIGURE 5.16

Oral cancer study. Aalen-Johansen and reverse Kaplan-Meier calculated in the test set patients. The gray lines in the left panel indicate the predicted risk of the null model at the 3-year prediction time horizon. The gray lines in the right panel show that 18.3% of the patients were lost to follow-up without event during the first 3 years on active surveillance.

cause-specific Cox regression models for the hazard rates of cancer progression and death without cancer progression, respectively, and extract the predicted 3-year risks of cancer progression. The hazard ratios of the two Cox regression models are shown in Table 5.4.1.

From this model, we extract the predicted 3-year risks of cancer progression in the test set of the active surveillance prostate cancer study. Figure 5.18 shows that many of the patients who experience cancer progression within 3 years receive a relatively high predicted risk, and most patients who either die due to other reasons within 3 years or stay alive and progression free during the first 3 years receive a relatively low predicted risk.

5.4.2   Brier score with competing risks

In the presence of competing risks, the weighted estimate of the average Brier score is obtained in the same manner as in the case without competing risks (Section 5.3.2). Now the test set data are divided into at least four groups with respect to a given prediction time horizon:

- Group *event*: contains all subjects who experience the event before the prediction time horizon.

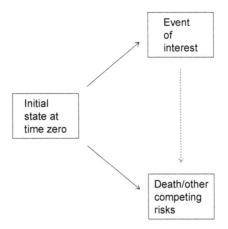

FIGURE 5.17
Multi-state model for survival analysis with competing risks. All subjects will either first experience the "Event of interest" or die or another of the "Competing risks" without the event of interest. In settings where the "Event of interest" is not fatal, subjects may experience "Competing risks" later on, but in the competing risks setting, this is not of interest. Censoring means that, for some subjects, the follow-up time is not long enough to observe the event and the event time.

TABLE 5.8
Active surveillance prostate cancer study. Results of cause-specific Cox regression. The Cox regression model for the hazard rate of progression of cancer uses 3 predictor variables and the Cox regression model for the hazard rate of death without progression uses only age.

Variable	Units	HazardRatio	CI.95	p-value
Cause: progression of cancer				
psa		1.17	[0.89; 1.56]	0.266
$ct1$	$cT1$	Ref		
	$cT2$	1.75	[0.78; 3.93]	0.177
diaggs	GNA	Ref		
	$3and3$	0.81	[0.36; 1.83]	0.617
	$3and4$	1.62	[0.60; 4.41]	0.341
Death without progression				
age		1.05	[0.95; 1.15]	0.344

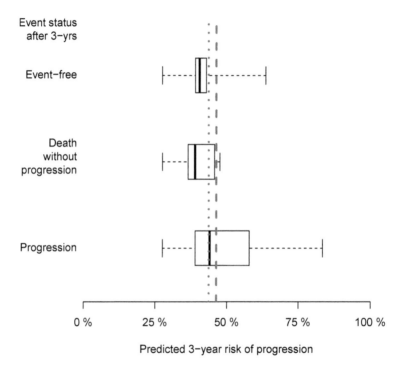

FIGURE 5.18
Active surveillance prostate cancer study. Boxplots showing the predicted 3-year risks of cancer progression (combined cause-specific Cox regression models) conditional on the outcome status after 3 years in the test set patients. The vertical dashed line is the Aalen-Johansen estimate in the test dataset and the vertical dotted line is the average of the combined cause-specific Cox model's risk predictions in the test dataset.

- Group *competing risks*: contains all subjects who experience a competing risk before the prediction time horizon.

- Group *event-free*: contains all subjects who were followed without the event until the prediction time horizon.

- Group *censored*: contains all subjects that are lost to follow-up before the prediction time horizon.

It is possible and sometimes useful to distinguish multiple competing risks. For example, in a study of intensive care unit (ICU) patients, discharge from the ICU and death are both competing risks for the event *hospital acquired infection*. Note that patients who experience an event or a competing risk after the prediction time horizon are in the *event-free* group.

To obtain the estimate of the average Brier score in the test set data, we calculate the squared distance for the subjects in the groups where the event status at the prediction time horizon is known (groups *event, competing risks,* and *event-free*). Instead of a simple average, we calculate a weighted average very much in the same way as described in Section 5.3.2, but now using the reverse Kaplan-Meier estimate of censoring (Figure 5.16, Panel B) to calculate the weights. The weights attached to subjects belonging to the *event* and the *competing risks* groups are evaluated at their individual event times, whereas the weights in the *event-free* group get weights that are evaluated at the prediction time horizon.

Thus, the calculation of the event-specific Brier score in the situation with competing risks and right-censored data needs almost no modification from the censored survival setting. But, there are at least two important differences. First, in the presence of competing risks and censored data, the Kaplan-Meier method is inappropriate for the absolute risk distribution. Hence, to obtain the benchmark null model which predicts the same risk to all subjects, we now use the Aalen-Johansen method [1]. The Aalen-Johansen method calculates the event-specific cumulative incidence in the test set data at the prediction time horizon. The second important difference is that one can, in principle, also predict the competing risks and the corresponding Brier scores. In the prostate cancer dataset, the competing risk is death due to reasons other than cancer, without cancer progression. This is not easy to interpret for the patient. Instead, one could either study prediction of the risk of the combined endpoint (progression or death due to any cause) or study the risk of all-cause mortality. Here, we simply predict the risk of cancer progression based on the cause-specific Cox regression models shown in Table 5.4.1 and calculate the Brier score in the test set of the active surveillance prostate cancer study.

```
# R-code
fit <- CSC(list(Hist(asprogtime,asprog)~psa+ct1+diaggs,
          Hist(asprogtime,asprog)~age),
        data=astrain,cause="progression")
Score(list("CSC"=fit),
```

```
data=astest,
formula=Hist(asprogtime,asprog)~1,
times=3,
metrics="brier",
cause="progression")
```

The Brier score of the model is lower, but not significantly lower, than the Brier score of the null model. This indicates that the model may have some predictive power, but the sample size is not large enough, or the predictor variables not strong enough, to make a significant difference.

5.4.3   Time-dependent AUC for competing risks

In the case with competing risks, the study of the discriminative ability of a risk prediction model is more challenging. Again, we are using the area under the time-dependent ROC curve. However, in the competing risks setting, the interpretation of the AUC needs to be modified compared to the binary setting because the group of patients without the event of interest is now a mixture of patients who experience the competing risk (e.g., death) and those who are alive and event-free at the prediction time horizon. Thus, the interpretation of the AUC is as follows: For a randomly chosen pair of subjects, where one subject has the event of interest before the prediction time horizon and the other has either experienced a competing risk or was event-free until the prediction time horizon, the concordance index (AUC) is the probability that the model assigns the higher risk to the subject who has experienced the event of interest.

As with the Brier score, the inverse probability of censoring weights can be obtained with the reverse Kaplan-Meier estimate (Figure 5.16, Panel B) [24]. In the active surveillance prostate cancer study we compute the AUC of the model that predicts the 3-year risks of cancer progression based on the Cox regression models shown in Table 5.4.1.

```
# R-code
fit <- CSC(list(Hist(asprogtime,asprog)~psa+ct1+diaggs,
       Hist(asprogtime,asprog)~age),
     data=astrain,cause="progression")
Score(list("CSC"=fit),data=astest,formula=Hist(asprogtime,asprog)~
    1,times=3,metrics="auc",cause="progression")
```

```
Metric AUC:

Results by model:

    model times  AUC lower upper
1:    CSC     3 62.8  49.3  76.2
```

```
NOTE: The higher AUC the better.
```

The AUC of the model is clearly above the 50% benchmark, indicating some discriminative power:

The probability is 62.8% that the model assigns the higher predicted risk to a patient who experiences progression of cancer within 3 years compared to a patient who either dies due to other reasons or is alive without progression after 3 years.

However, the confidence interval includes the 50% benchmark indicating that the sample size is not large enough or the predictor variables not strong enough to make a difference. The corresponding ROC curves for the predicted 3-year risks of cancer progression are obtained as follows:

```
# R-code
fit <- CSC(list(Hist(asprogtime,asprog)~psa+ct1+diaggs,
        Hist(asprogtime,asprog)~age),
        data=astrain,cause="progression")
x <- Score(list("CSC"=fit),
        data=astest,
        formula=Hist(asprogtime,asprog)~1,
        times=3,
        metrics="auc",
        plots="ROC",
        cause="progression")
plotROC(x,plot.main="Outcome: 3 year cancer progression")
```

The resulting ROC curve is shown in Figure 5.19.

5.4.4 Calibration curve for competing risks

In order to calculate the calibration curve of a prediction model in a situation with competing risks, the only difference from the censored survival case is that the observed frequency of the outcome is calculated with the Aalen-Johansen method instead of the Kaplan-Meier method. Also, when pseudo-values are used, these are calculated with the Aalen-Johansen method [77]. The pseudo-value approach works under the assumption that the censoring mechanism is completely independent of the covariates and the outcome. This assumption is relaxed when we calculate the observed frequency at predicted risk p locally in the subgroup of patients who received a predicted risk close to p. This local estimate is obtained with the option /cens.method = "local"/in the R-code below. The estimate of the calibration curve which is based on pseudo-values is obtained by setting the option *cens.method = "pseudo"* instead.

In the active surveillance prostate cancer study, the calibration curves for the prediction model which combines cause-specific Cox regressions models to predict the 3-year risks of cancer progression is obtained as follows:

```
# R-code
fit <- CSC(list(Hist(asprogtime,asprog)~psa+ct1+diaggs,
```

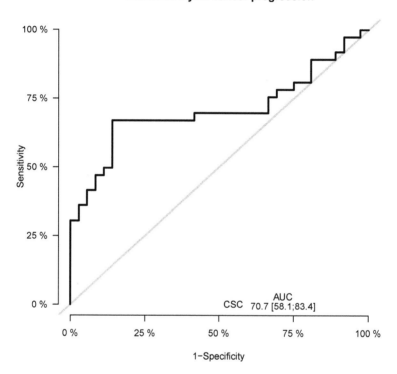

FIGURE 5.19
Active surveillance prostate cancer study. ROC curve for a prediction model which combines two cause-specific Cox regression models to predict the 3-year risks of cancer progression accounting for the competing risk of mortality unrelated to cancer in the test set.

```
        Hist(asprogtime,asprog)~age),
        data=astrain,cause="progression")
x <- Score(list("CSC"=fit), data=astest,
        formula=Hist(asprogtime,asprog)~1, times=3,
        plots="calibration", cause="progression")
plotCalibration(x,cens.method="local")
```

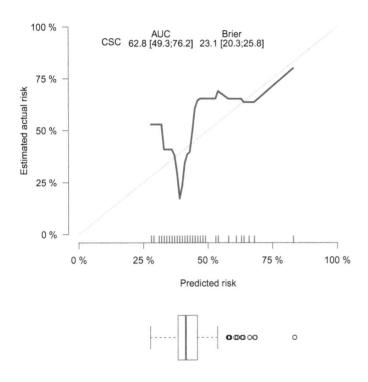

FIGURE 5.20

Active surveillance prostate cancer study. Calibration curve for a prediction model which combines two cause-specific Cox regression models to predict the 3-year risk of cancer progression in the presence of the competing risk of mortality unrelated to cancer. The rug plot at the bottom and the boxplot below show the distribution of the predicted 3-year risk of cancer progression.

The calibration curve shown in Figure 5.20 indicates that the model is not perfectly calibrated because, in the region where there are many of the predicted 3-year risks close to 40% risk (indicated by the rug plot and the boxplot), the curve deviates considerably from the diagonal. This may be due to weak signal in the predictor variables, misspecification of the model, or a relatively small sample size. Salvation for the calibration of this particular model could, for example, be obtained with shrinkage or other means of penalized likelihood (See Section 8.2.1). Figure 5.21 shows that a similar pattern of miscalibration is present for earlier and later prediction time horizons. The figure also shows that the location of most of the predicted risks increases (as it should) when the prediction time horizon is increased.

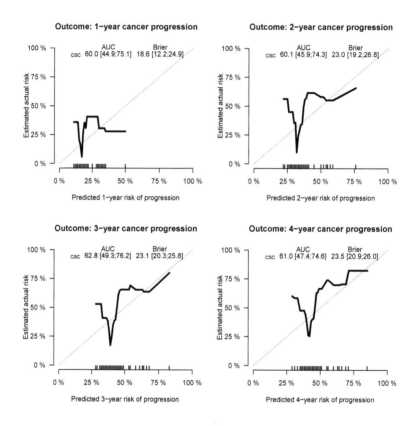

FIGURE 5.21
Active surveillance prostate cancer study. Calibration curves for varying prediction time horizons for a prediction model that combines two cause-specific Cox regression models to predict the risks of cancer progression in the presence of the competing risk of mortality unrelated to cancer.

5.5 The Index of Prediction Accuracy (IPA)

While there are many metrics for predictive accuracy proposed in the literature, many of them are either not intuitive or not proper. For this reason, we have restricted coverage to measures such as the area under the ROC curve and the Brier score. A concern with the first measure is that it reflects only discrimination. Also, it does not distinguish between a useless prediction model and a harmful one. A useless model, for example, might predict a random number between 0 and 1. A model that randomly predicts 0s and 1s may indeed be useless but it may also be harmful since it suggests certainty in its predictions. A risk prediction model is deemed harmful when it is outperformed by the benchmark null model (the best of the useless models) which ignores the predictor variables and predicts the same risk to all patients.

The Brier score reflects both discrimination and calibration. However, the values of the Brier score are on a scale which does not allow unconditional interpretation. To interpret the value of the Brier score we need to know the Brier score of the benchmark null model which in turn depends on the situation at hand (Figure 5.4). To interpret the performance of a model we calculate the Index of Prediction Accuracy (IPA) [115] which is obtained very much in the same way as the explained variation index R^2 for linear regression; it is one minus the ratio of the model Brier score to the null model Brier score [82]. The main difference to many other R^2 measures is that, to calculate the IPA, we either use an external test dataset or some form of cross-validation (Sections 2.6.2, 7.4). The IPA reflects both discrimination and calibration as well as distinguishes useless models (IPA=0) from harmful models (IPA< 0). The IPA can be used in binary, time-to-event, and competing risks settings. Also, extensions to time dynamic prediction models and landmark analysis are readily available [68, 137].

The IPA is obtained in any of the three settings (binary, time-to-event, and competing risks) by adding the option *summary = "ipa"* as illustrated below for the example of our active surveillance prostate cancer study

```
# R-code
fit <- CSC(list(Hist(asprogtime,asprog)~psa+ct1+diaggs,
        Hist(asprogtime,asprog)~age),
    data=astrain,cause="progression")
x <- Score(list("CSC"=fit),cause="progression",contrasts=FALSE,
    data=astest, formula=Hist(asprogtime,asprog)~1,
    times=3, summary="ipa",metrics="brier")
x
```

Metric Brier:

Results by model:

```
model times Brier lower upper IPA
1: Null model    3  24.9  23.2  26.6 0.0
2:        CSC    3  23.1  20.3  25.8 7.1
```

NOTE: The lower Brier the better, the higher IPA the better.

5.6   Choice of prediction time horizon

In right-censored data, with or without competing risks, one has to choose a prediction time horizon within the maximum follow-up period of both the training and the test data such that it is possible to predict the risks based on the training data and to estimate the prediction performance parameters in the test data.

> *The machine learning mindset yields a useful rule of thumb for limiting the maximum value of the prediction time horizon.*

It may be difficult to come up with general rules on how to do this because the best choice will always depend on the subject matter question. However, limitations of the available data, and here in particular limited follow-up, should also be considered.

A useful rule of thumb for the maximum allowed prediction time horizon comes from the machine learning way of thinking: do not use a prediction time horizon value so large that you get error messages in either the model fitting or the model evaluation steps under data perturbation. One way to do this is to draw many bootstrap datasets (Section 2.6.6) from our training dataset. We then collect the values of the maximum follow-up times of the individual bootstrap datasets and determine their minimum. This yields an initial upper bound for the prediction time horizon. Indeed, most modeling techniques, including Cox regression, will produce an error when you try to predict the event risk at a time point beyond the maximum follow-up time in the data. In the process of cross-validation (Section 7.4), it may however still happen that either one of the modeling algorithms or the estimate of the prediction performance fails when few subjects are followed up and are at risk of the event at the prediction time horizon. Then, one should consider analyzing an earlier prediction time horizon.

5.7 Time-dependent prediction performance

In some applications it is difficult to specify a single prediction horizon; in others, it may be of interest to consider multiple prediction time horizons. It is easy enough to repeat the computation of the Brier score, IPA and AUC for multiple time points, but beware of cherry-picking. Useful graphs are then obtained by plotting the results against the time of the prediction time horizon. This is illustrated in our oral cancer study where Figure 5.22 is obtained with the following R-code:

```
# R-code
fit <- coxph(Surv(survtime,survstatus)~age+tumorthickness+grade,
        data=octrain, x=1L)
x <- Score(list("Cox"=fit),
        data=octest, formula=Surv(survtime,survstatus)~1,
        times=seq(12,120,12), se.fit=0, contrasts=FALSE,
        summary="ipa", contrast=FALSE)
```

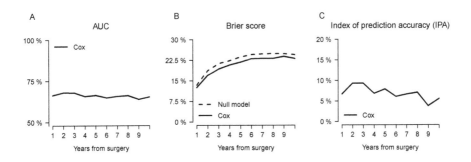

FIGURE 5.22
Oral cancer study. Time-dependent AUC (panel A), time-dependent Brier score (Panel B) and time-dependent IPA (Panel C) of a Cox regression model which was fitted in the learning set. Performance metrics are calculated in the validation set.

6

How do I decide between rival models?

You are here because you want to compare different statistical methods. Or, you want to assess the effect of adding a new source of predictors (new markers) to an existing prediction model. Sometimes there is an established prediction model and you want to see if a new model that you just made predicts any better. Alternatively, you may have come across two published prediction models that predict the same outcome and both are applicable to your patients; here you would like to know which one would be more accurate in your patients. Thus, we have the situation where there are (at least) two models available that both predict the risk of an event for individual patients. In this chapter, we assume the case where an independent test dataset is available for the comparison of models. Please refer to Chapter 7.4 to see examples of the case where the models have to be built and validated using a single dataset.

When comparing rival models, one of them might be more expensive (i.e., require inputs such as a costly blood test) or more invasive (require a biopsy rather than only a blood draw), either of which would suggest that a small drop in accuracy might outweigh the cost or pain of running the other model. In other words, there could be a trade-off between accuracy and cost/invasiveness. To simplify the situation here, let us assume that is not the case, and we would simply prefer the more accurate model, such that the focus here is solely on accuracy. The goal is to decide which model would be more accurate in prospective patients. It is not uncommon to see a situation in which a model is currently in use in clinical practice, and a new model has been developed with the aim to improve the risk predictions. Here the question is whether we should switch to the new model. We would only want to do this if it is substantially more accurate, since the old model is trusted by the medical community and already embedded in their workflow. An example of this is the PCPT risk calculator for prostate cancer [10]. This calculator was getting considerable use, with many thousands of hits per week for the online risk calculator. However, the approach to biopsy recently changed, among other things, leading to a consortium who combined their data to make a new model (the PBCG risk calculator) [11]. The new model was found to be more accurate than the standby PCPT. The argument for switching to PBCG was solely based on the improved accuracy, especially since there was friction in the medical community with respect to moving away from the trusted PCPT calculator.

6.1 Model comparison roadmap

The tools for model comparison begin with those described in the roadmap for individual model evaluation, as specified in Section 5.1. We plot predicted probabilities, calculate the performance metrics (Brier score, AUC, IPA) and plot the calibrations of rival models. This is applicable whether the rival models are

- a new model (experimental model) being compared with an existing model (conventional model),

- various new models being compared with one another, or

- the evaluation of a new marker in a model, versus the model, which lacks the new marker.

We then turn our attention to the difference in prediction performance between two rival models, measured by the difference in the AUC and Brier score. Since each individual subject receives predictions from each of the rival models, this setting is analogous to that of a paired t-test (Brier score) or of a signed-rank test/paired Wilcoxon test (AUC), where the test of the difference can be statistically significant yet the confidence intervals for the individual metrics overlap. Scatterplots showing the predicted risks of one model on the x-axis and of the other model on the y-axis are insightful descriptive statistics. If the plot shows a lot of change, i.e., points away from the 45-degree line, this implies a potentially substantial impact from switching from one risk prediction model to another.

6.2 Analysis of rival prediction models

In order to determine which model predicts more accurately on average, we consider the performance metrics described in Chapter 5. Now it is time to compute differences between these metrics for two rival models to determine which model is better on average and by what magnitude. We also provide confidence intervals as well as tests of significance for the differences of the Brier scores and AUCs, respectively. As in the previous chapters, we discuss the three settings (uncensored, censored without competing risks, censored with competing risks) and illustrate the learning and test datasets of the three applications (in vitro fertilization study, oral cancer study, active surveillance prostate cancer study).

6.2.1   Uncensored binary outcome

In our in vitro fertilization study, for the purpose of illustration, suppose our subject matter experts suggested a conventional logistic regression model which includes additive effects of the number of antral follicles, the smoking status, the cycle length and the age of the woman. Table 5.2 shows the odds ratios of this model. We next construct an experimental model to see if its performance would be superior to the conventional model in prediction performance. Compared to the conventional model, the experimental model includes three more variables (FSH, BMI, ovarian volume) and describes the effect of the number of antral follicles with a restricted cubic spline that is further allowed to interact with smoking status. The interaction yields a possibly modified effect as the model allows the relationship between the risk of ovarian hyperstimulation syndrome and the number of antral follicles to be different in smokers than in non-smokers. To avoid overfitting we also add a ridge penalty term; however, we do not optimize its value (see Chapter 8.2.1). The following R-code shows how we fit the two logistic regression models in the training dataset and evaluate the performance in the test dataset.

```
# R-code
# conventional model
fit1 <- lrm(ohss~ant.foll+cyclelen+smoking+age,data=ivftrain)
# experimental model
fit2 <- lrm(ohss~rcs(ant.foll,3)*smoking+cyclelen+age+fsh+bmi+
    ovolume,data=ivftrain,penalty=10)
# head to head comparison in test dataset
x <- Score(list("Conventional"=fit1,"Experimental"=fit2),
    data=ivftest, formula=ohss~1, summary=c("risks","ipa"),
    plots=c("roc","cal"))
# scatterplot showing predicted risks of the rival models
plotRisk(x,
    col=c("gray22","black"),
    xlab="Conventional model: risk of OHSS",
    ylab="Experimental model: risk of OHSS")
```

Figure 6.1 shows that compared to the conventional model, the experimental model predicts generally higher risks in test set patients with low predicted risks (below 25% risk) and generally lower risks in the test set patients with high risks (above 25% risks). Considering the symbols that indicate the observed outcome of the test set patients, the scatterplot suggests that the experimental model has lower prediction accuracy when compared to the conventional model. This is because many of the subjects who receive a higher predicted risk by the experimental model did not have ovarian hyperstimulation syndrome and many of the subjects who receive a lower predicted risk by the experimental model did have ovarian hyperstimulation syndrome. Hence, it seems that switching to the experimental model would be a move in the wrong direction. However, it is not recommended to simply read off such a conclusion from the scatterplot, because in fact there may be dots on top of dots, and because we have more appropriate metrics to summarize what we see.

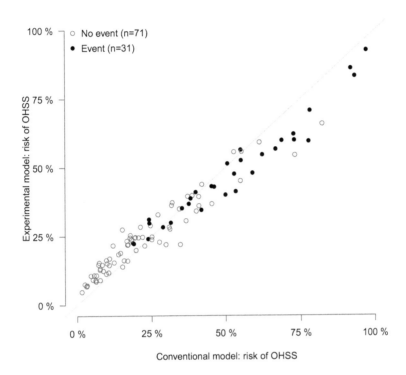

FIGURE 6.1
In vitro fertilization study. Scatterplot of risk predictions from conventional model versus experimental model.

Table 6.1 shows that the experimental model has the slightly higher AUC than the conventional model. However, it appears that the calibration of the conventional model is much better. This is seen by comparing the Brier scores (the lower the better) and the corresponding IPAs (the higher the better). The following code produces Table 6.1.

```
# R-code
summary(x,what="score")
```

Table 6.2 zooms in on the overall performance differences of the models. Although we see that the differences shown in Table 6.2 are identical to the difference in means in Table 6.1, the analysis of differences is necessary to get

TABLE 6.1

In vitro fertilization study. Test set results for the AUC, Brier score and IPA
for the null model, the conventional model and the experimental model.

Model	AUC	Brier (%)	IPA
Null model	50.0	21.2 [17.6;24.7]	0.0
Conventional	86.5 [79.5;93.5]	14.0 [10.5;17.4]	34.1
Experimental	86.9 [80.0;93.8]	14.6 [11.5;17.6]	31.2

accurate standard errors. For the Brier score residuals, these are calculated
very much in the same way as for a paired t-test (i.e., one-sample t-test).
The data are paired because each patient in the test dataset receive two risk
predictions, one from each model. The standard error for the difference in
the AUC is obtained by the Delong-Delong method [52]. The following code
produces Table 6.2.

```
# R-code
summary(x,what="contrasts")
```

TABLE 6.2

In vitro fertilization study. Test set results comparing the experimental model
(Exp.) with the conventional model (Conv.) in terms of differences of prediction performance.

Model	Reference	Δ AUC (%)	p-value	Δ Brier (%)	p-value
Exp.	Conv.	0.41 [-1.76;2.58]	0.71	0.60 [-0.42;1.62]	0.25

To get a full picture of what is going on, we now look at the calibration
plot in Figure 6.2. The calibration plot is obtained with the R-code:

```
# R-code
plotCalibration(x,auc.in.legend=1,brier.in.legend=1)
```

The slight benefit in the AUC of the experimental model is overwhelmed by its
less optimal calibration as evidenced by the increased departure from the 45-
degree line compared to the conventional model. The net result of the increase
in the AUC yet decrease in calibration is an increased Brier score. In other
words, the Brier score reflects both discrimination and calibration. The results
suggest that when you consider both aspects of prediction performance, the
experimental model fares worse.

In a situation like this, it is useful to consider the possible explanations for
the findings. One possible explanation is that the additional features are truly
not helpful. Another explanation is that, although one or more of the additional features are helpful, the role of a helpful feature is not correctly specified

or not correctly learned from the specific training dataset, or disturbed by an unhelpful feature. Note that in our example the size of the training dataset is rather small. The AUC and the Brier score have been criticized for being insensitive to detecting predictor variable signals [140]. Our example here illustrates that, for a variety of reasons, this may not be the case. We have listed several reasons why the AUC did not improve by much and why the Brier score may have gotten worse.

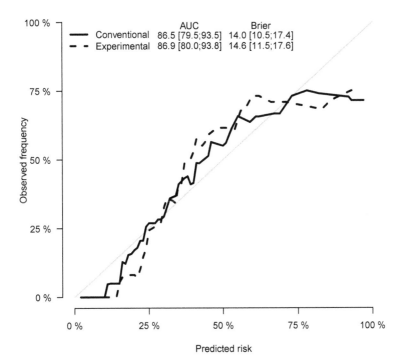

FIGURE 6.2
In vitro fertilization study. Calibration plots of conventional and experimental models.

Figure 6.3 shows overlayed ROC curves for the two models. These are obtained with the R-code:

```
# R-code
plotROC(x)
```

In this example, the display is not terribly helpful. For one thing, one should not use the ROC curve to decide the cut-point if the prediction was going to be categorized as positive or negative. The determination of the optimal cut-point is more complicated and involves a medical decision to be made, and corresponding utility and costs. For another reason, the reader may be tempted to choose a cut-point that maximizes the deviation between two models. Again this decision would not appropriately consider utility and costs or other outcomes.

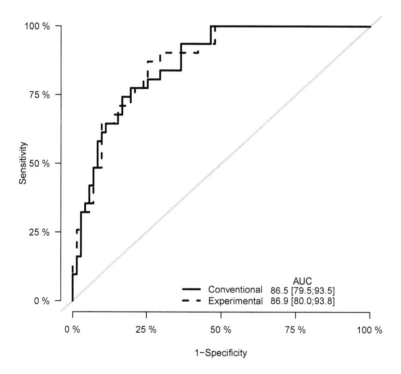

FIGURE 6.3
In vitro fertilization study. ROC curves for conventional and experimental models.

6.2.2 Right-censored time-to-event outcome (without competing risks)

In the setting with a right-censored time-to-event outcome, we must choose one or several prediction time horizon values (Section 5.6). At each prediction time horizon, we can compare the predictive performance of rival models. We can also display the comparative performance as a function of the prediction time horizon. The other main characteristic of this setting is censoring. We deal with censored data in the way we described in Chapter 5. Finally, before building and comparing models, one needs to somehow deal with missing values in the predictor variables. To illustrate the right-censored outcome scenario, we thus restrict the training and test sets of the oral cancer study to the complete cases (with respect to the predictor variables used below).

In the oral cancer study, for the purpose of illustration, the conventional model is a Cox regression model. Fitting the Cox regression model to the training set produces the nomogram shown in Figure 6.4.

```
# R-code
dd <- datadist(octrain.cc)
options(datadist="dd")
fit1 <- cph(Surv(survtime,survstatus)~rcs(age,3)+rcs(tumorthickness
    ,3)+gender+tobacco+deep.invasion+site+race+x.posnodes+
    tumormaxdimension+vascular.invasion,data=octrain.cc,x=TRUE,surv
    =TRUE)
surv <- Survival(fit1)
plot(nomogram(fit1,fun=list(function(x) 1-surv(60, x),
            function(x) 1-surv(120, x)),
        funlabel=c("5 year risk","10 year risk")))
```

Suppose that the subject matter experts stated that all the variables shown in Figure 6.4 should be included. Our experimental model uses the same variables but a more flexible modeling technique, the random survival forest [102]. The experimental model is obtained with the following R-code:

```
# R-code
set.seed(1972)
fit2 <- rfsrc(Surv(survtime,survstatus)~ age+tumorthickness+gender+
    tobacco+deep.invasion+site+race+x.posnodes+tumormaxdimension+
    vascular.invasion,data=octrain.cc)
```

Note that we set the random seed to be able to reproduce the exact same random forest model when the code is re-executed.

Based on both models, we can predict at any prediction time horizon value up to 20 years. This is because the patient of the training dataset with the longest follow-up time was followed for 20 years (Figure 4.1). For the purpose of illustration we show results at prediction time horizon values of 1, 5, 10, and 15 years. In Table 6.3 we see that the experimental model outperforms the conventional model at all prediction time horizons on all metrics. The following R-code produces Table 6.3:

```
# R-code
fit1 <- cph(Surv(survtime,survstatus)~rcs(age,3)+tumorthickness+
    gender+tobacco+deep.invasion+site+race+x.posnodes+
    tumormaxdimension+vascular.invasion,
```

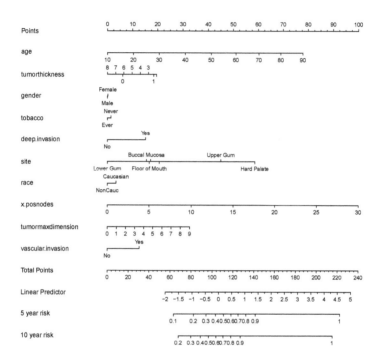

FIGURE 6.4

Oral cancer study. Nomogram illustrating the Cox regression model used as a conventional model. The model predicts all-cause mortality risks based on values for the predictor variables for any given prediction time horizon. The 5-year and 10-year prediction time horizons are selected for illustration. See Section 4.6.5 for how to read a nomogram.

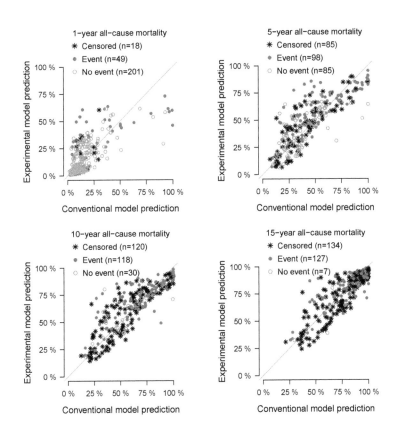

FIGURE 6.5

Oral cancer study. Scatterplots of the conventional (Cox regression) versus the experimental model (random survival forest) predictions at 1-, 5-, 10-, and 15-year prediction time horizons.

```
                data=octrain.cc, x=TRUE, y=TRUE, surv=TRUE)
set.seed(1972)
fit2 <- rfsrc(Surv(survtime,survstatus)~ age+tumorthickness+gender+
    tobacco+deep.invasion+site+race+x.posnodes+tumormaxdimension+
    vascular.invasion,data=octrain.cc)
x <- Score(list("Conventional"=fit1,"Experimental"=fit2),
        data=octest.cc,
        formula=Surv(survtime,survstatus)~1,
        times=c(12,60,120,180),
        summary=c("risks","IPA"),
        plots=c("cali","roc"))
summary(x,what="score")[[1]]
```

However, the improvement is statistically significant for only the 1-year and the 5-year prediction time horizons (see Table 6.4). Table 6.4 is produced with the following R-code:

```
# R-code
summary(x,what="contrasts")
```

At the 1-year, 5-year and 10-year prediction time horizons the experimental model has higher discriminative performance than the conventional model and it is also well-calibrated (Figure 6.7). This performance advantage of the experimental model appears to be quite stable across the prediction time horizons (Figures 6.8 and 6.9). For whatever reason, the prediction performances of the two models are more comparable at the 15-year prediction time horizon, despite the fact that the predicted risks themselves remain different (Figure 6.5). There are a number of reasons that a forest model might outperform a Cox regression model. One is that the proportional hazard assumption of the Cox regression model might not be appropriate in this setting. Another issue is that important interaction terms might be needed, and these were left unspecified in our conventional model. The forest can represent both interactions and non-linear relationships more flexibly than can our conventional Cox regression model.

We should note that moving the prediction time horizon beyond 15 years is possible but questionable. There are only very few test set patients (with no missing values in the predictor variables) at risk after 15 years (see Figure 6.6). This means that our way of estimating performance parameters is unreliable at later prediction time horizons. We rely on inverse probability weights which yield unstable estimates when the number at risk gets small. In reality, you cannot use the maximum follow-up time in your dataset as the prediction time horizon (see Section 5.6).

In the training set of our oral cancer study the minimum time across 100,000 bootstrap samples turns out to be 13.83 years which is clearly below 20 years.

```
# R-code
library(bootstrap)
```

```
set.seed(8)
# time of death or censored in the complete cases
# of the training set
boot.max <- bootstrap(octrain.cc$survtime,
            100000, # number of bootstrap samples
            theta=function(x){max(x)}) # maximum time
# minimum of the bootstrap maxima, divided by 12
# to convert from months to years
min(boot.max$thetastar)/12
```

[1] 13.83333

Thus, with this rule of thumb, a prediction time horizon beyond 13.83 years should not be used. Note that we picked this very large number of bootstrap repetitions to avoid a random seed effect.

TABLE 6.3
Oral cancer study. Test set results for the AUC, Brier score and IPA at 1, 5, 10, and 15 year prediction time horizons.

Years	Model	AUC (%)	Brier (%)	IPA
1	Null model	50.0	15.4 [10.3;20.5]	0.0
1	Conventional	69.1 [59.8;78.4]	13.9 [9.2;18.6]	10.0
1	Experimental	78.6 [70.7;86.6]	12.1 [8.2;16.0]	21.3
5	Null model	50.0	24.4 [21.0;27.9]	0.0
5	Conventional	73.0 [65.8;80.2]	20.6 [16.7;24.4]	15.8
5	Experimental	80.6 [74.4;86.8]	18.2 [15.1;21.3]	25.5
10	Null model	50.0	23.6 [21.0;26.2]	0.0
10	Conventional	65.9 [55.7;76.2]	23.1 [19.0;27.2]	2.0
10	Experimental	71.1 [61.8;80.4]	21.3 [17.8;24.7]	9.9
15	Null model	50.0	16.6 [10.9;22.3]	0.0
15	Conventional	78.5 [65.7;91.3]	14.2 [8.9;19.5]	14.3
15	Experimental	82.2 [70.5;93.9]	13.3 [8.1;18.4]	20.0

To show how the prediction performance of the two models evolves, we plot the Brier score against time (Figure 6.8). The graph is obtained with the following code:

```
# R-code
x <- Score(list("Conventional"=fit1,"Experimental"=fit2),
      data=octest.cc,
      formula=Surv(survtime,survstatus)~1,
      times=seq(12,180,6))
plotBrier(x,
      legend.x="bottomleft",
      xlab="Years from surgery",
```

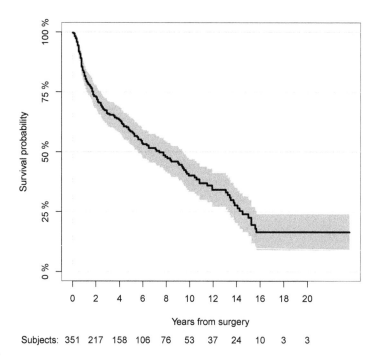

FIGURE 6.6
Oral cancer study. Kaplan-Meier estimate of overall survival in the subset
of the test set patients who had no missing values in any of the predictor
variables.

TABLE 6.4
Oral cancer study test set results. Shown are differences between the experimental model (Random survival forest) and the conventional model (Cox
regression) as Δ AUC and Δ Brier score at 1-, 5-, 10-, and 15-year prediction
time horizons.

Years	Model	Ref.	Δ AUC (%)	p-value	Δ Brier (%)	p-value
1	Exp.	Conv.	9.6 [2.1;17.1]	0.0125	-1.7 [-3.4;-0.1]	0.041
5	Exp.	Conv.	7.6 [2.7;12.4]	0.0022	-2.4 [-4.5;-0.2]	0.030
10	Exp.	Conv.	5.2 [-2.5;12.8]	0.1845	-1.8 [-4.6;0.9]	0.185
15	Exp.	Conv.	3.7 [-6.5;13.9]	0.4783	-0.9 [-3.7;1.8]	0.510

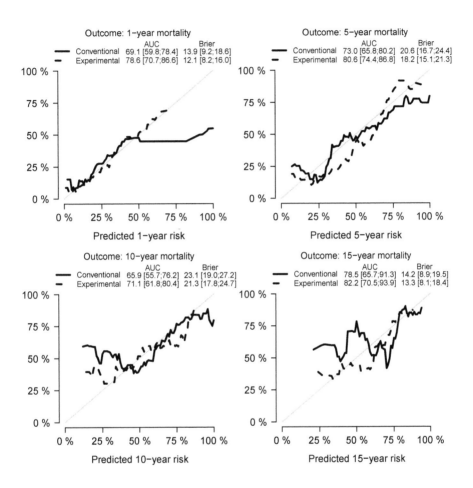

FIGURE 6.7

Oral cancer study. Calibration plots for the experimental model (Random survival forest) and conventional model (Cox regression) at different prediction time horizons.

```
        axis1.at=seq(0,180,12),
        axis1.labels=seq(0,15,1))
```

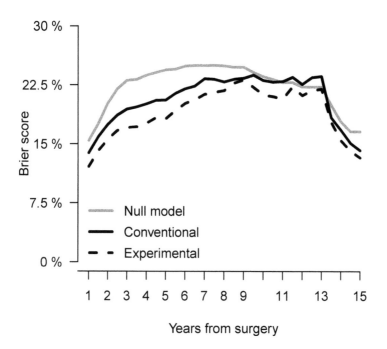

FIGURE 6.8
Oral cancer study. Shown are Brier scores as a function of horizon time, for
the null model, the conventional model, and the experimental model.

In the figure, we see that no matter the specific prediction time horizon
that is chosen, the experimental model is at least as accurate as or better than
the conventional model. Similarly, we plot the AUC against time (Figure 6.9).
Also here the experimental model discriminates better than the conventional
model, regardless of the prediction time horizon chosen. The graph is obtained
with the following code:

```
# R-code
x <- Score(list("Conventional"=fit1,"Experimental"=fit2),
      data=octest.cc,
      formula=Surv(survtime,survstatus)~1,
```

```
        times=seq(12,180,6))
plotAUC(x, legend.x="bottomleft",
    xlab="Years from surgery",
    lwd=3,lty=c(1,2),
    axis1.at=seq(0,180,12),
    axis1.labels=seq(0,15,1))
```

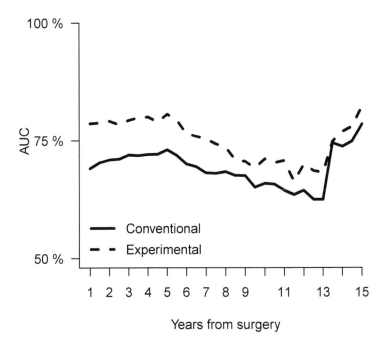

FIGURE 6.9
Oral cancer study. The AUC as a function of the prediction time horizon, for
the conventional and experimental models.

6.2.3 Competing risks

There are multiple methods to model competing risk data. The most common
approach is probably the use of the Fine-Gray regression model [66]. For
simplicity, we will build our conventional model using this approach. When it
comes to predicting the risk of an event in the presence of competing risks,

there is an alternative approach that relies upon cause-specific Cox regression models [17, 135]. We use this approach to build our experimental model.

For both approaches, one should include predictor variables that are believed to be associated with the event of interest or the competing risk. For example, in our active surveillance prostate cancer study we should include comorbidities such as cardiac disease or diabetes as they are associated with death unrelated to prostate cancer. Unfortunately, we do not have these variables in our datasets, but ideally, we would have included them.

The regression coefficients of our conventional and the experimental models fitted to the training dataset of our active surveillance prostate cancer study are shown in Tables 6.5 and 6.2.3, respectively.

```
# R-code
fit1 <- FGR(Hist(asprogtime,asprog)~age+psa+ct1+diaggs+ppb5,data=
    astrain,cause="progression")
fit1
```

TABLE 6.5

Active surveillance prostate cancer study. Regression coefficients (as subdistribution hazard ratios) of Fine-Gray regression model.

Variable	subHR	ci	p
age	0.9784	[0.91;1.05]	0.5200
psa	1.1958	[0.85;1.67]	0.3000
ct1cT2	1.4258	[0.57;3.56]	0.4500
diaggs3 and 3	0.8323	[0.37;1.87]	0.6600
diaggs3 and 4	1.6919	[0.67;4.27]	0.2700
ppb5	1.1225	[0.98;1.29]	0.1000

```
# R-code
fit2 <- CSC(list(Hist(asprogtime,asprog)~age+psa+ct1+diaggs+ppb5,
    Hist(asprogtime,asprog)~age),data=astrain,cause="progression")
fit2
```

Not surprisingly, the predicted risks from the cause-specific Cox regression models and the Fine-Gray regression model are quite similar for all test set patients. This is expected since both models are regression models with the same set of predictor variables, and it is nicely illustrated by a scatterplot showing the predicted 3-year risks of the rival models in Figure 6.10. The risk scatterplot is obtained with the following R-code:

```
# R-code
x <- Score(list("Conventional"=fit1,"Experimental"=fit2),
        data=astest,
        formula=Hist(asprogtime,asprog)~1,
        times=3,summary="risk",
```

TABLE 6.6
Active surveillance prostate cancer study. Results of cause-specific Cox regression. The Cox regression model for the hazard rate of the progression of cancer uses 5 predictor variables and the Cox regression model for the hazard rate of death without progression uses only age.

Variable	Units	HazardRatio	CI.95	p-value
		Cause: progression of cancer		
age		0.98	[0.92; 1.05]	0.6479
psa		1.20	[0.89; 1.61]	0.2330
ct1	cT1	Ref		
	cT2	1.45	[0.62; 3.41]	0.3919
diaggs	GNA	Ref		
	3and3	0.77	[0.34; 1.74]	0.5247
	3and4	1.58	[0.58; 4.32]	0.3724
ppb5		1.13	[0.99; 1.28]	0.0714
		Death without progression		
age		1.05	[0.95; 1.15]	0.344

```
          cause="progression")
   plotRisk(x,
        times=3,
        plot.main="Risk of progression within 3 years",
        xlab="Conventional model prediction",
        ylab="Experimental model prediction")
```

TABLE 6.7
Active surveillance prostate cancer study. Test set results. Prediction performance at 3-year prediction time horizon of the conventional model (Fine-Gray regression) and the experimental model (cause-specific Cox regression).

Years	Model	AUC (%)	Brier (%)	IPA
3	Null model	50.0	24.9 [23.2;26.6]	0.0
3	Conventional	70.1 [57.4;82.7]	21.5 [18.6;24.4]	13.7
3	Experimental	70.7 [58.1;83.4]	21.2 [18.4;24.1]	14.6

Since this is the case, it is not surprising to see that the performance metrics are also very similar (Table 6.7). For all practical purposes, these two models are interchangeable. The following R-code produces Table 6.7:

```
# R-code
x <- Score(list("Conventional"=fit1,"Experimental"=fit2),
      data=astest,
      formula=Hist(asprogtime,asprog)~1,
```

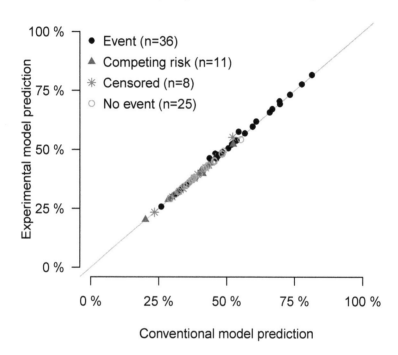

FIGURE 6.10
Active surveillance prostate cancer study. Scatterplot of the predicted risks of
cancer progression from the conventional model (Fine-Gray regression) and
the experimental model (cause-specific Cox regression).

```
        times=3,
        cause="progression")
summary(x,what="score")
```

Hypothetically, if we had to move one of these models forward into production, we would favor the experimental model, since it had a significantly better Brier score (see Table 6.8). The table is obtained as follows:

```
# R-code
summary(x,what="contrasts")
```

TABLE 6.8
Active surveillance prostate cancer study test set results. Shown are differences between the experimental model (cause-specific Cox regression) and the conventional model (Fine-Gray regression) as Δ AUC and Δ Brier score at the 3 year prediction time horizon.

Years	Model	Ref.	Δ AUC (%)	p-value	Δ Brier (%)	p-value
3	Exp.	Conv.	0.64 [-0.08;1.36]	0.084	-0.21 [-0.36;-0.07]	0.004

In addition, the experimental model had a slightly higher AUC and a slightly lower Brier score across all time points (Figures 6.12 and 6.11).

```
# R-code
x <- Score(list("Conventional"=fit1,"Experimental"=fit2),
        data=astest, formula=Hist(asprogtime,asprog)~1,
        cause="progression", times=seq(.5,5,.5))
plotBrier(x)
plotAUC(x)
```

However, examination of the calibration curve at the 3-year prediction time horizon deserves special attention (Figure 6.13). First off, both models have calibration issues with somewhat serious departures from the 45-degree line. Secondly, each model has slightly better calibration than the other one in separate parts of the curve. However, the experimental model trumps the conventional model in regions of the risk scale where most of the risk predictions are.

6.3 Clinically relevant change of prediction

As specified in our roadmap, we use performance metrics to choose which prediction model is preferred, but these metrics do not fully tell us what choice

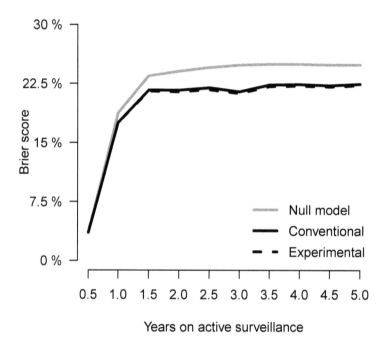

FIGURE 6.11
Active surveillance prostate cancer study test set results. Brier score as a
function of the horizon time for the null model, the conventional model (Fine-
Gray regression), and the experimental model (cause-specific Cox regression).

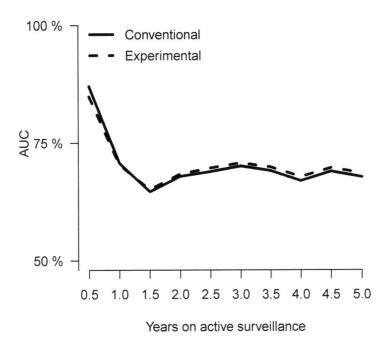

FIGURE 6.12
Active surveillance prostate cancer study test set results. The AUC as a function of the horizon time for the null model, the conventional model (Fine-Gray regression), and the experimental model (cause-specific Cox regression).

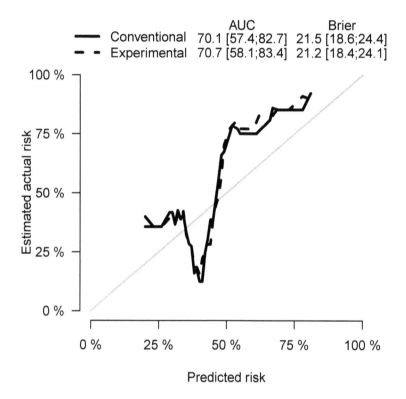

FIGURE 6.13
Active surveillance prostate cancer study. Calibration plot showing the conventional model (Fine-Gray regression) and the experimental model (cause-specific Cox regression).

to make (i.e., Model A vs Model B). The improvement in performance (e.g., IPA or AUC) must be judged in the context of the degree of differences in the predicted risks, since changing models (e.g., from A to B) involves effort and cost (e.g., programming and clinical training). Therefore, we have recommended in our roadmap that a clinical expert help define what change in predicted probability is noteworthy, since a change in predicted probability from a model is easier for someone to interpret than is a change in a performance metric like the AUC. The clinical expert can help to judge whether a 10% predicted probability is different from a 20% predicted probability, and we have developed a process to conduct this assessment.

The first step is to consider having a subject matter expert help you outline a region of clinically significant change. Begin by plotting an empty two-dimensional space with risk from one model on the x-axis and the risk from the other model on the y-axis. The axes are probabilities of the event. The concept here is to define the region within which the risk difference between the models is not clinically interesting. For example, the area near the 45-degree line will typically not be clinically interesting and therefore define the region of meaningless change. For an example of the clinically (un)interesting area, see Panel A of Figure 6.14. In the figure the elliptical region around the 45-degree line is not shaded and therefore indicates an area of meaningless risk difference. If the conventional model predicts 43% risk for a new patient while the on-average more accurate experimental model predicts 43.8% for the same patient, then this difference would not lead to different clinical decisions as indicated by the non-shaded region. Generally, the off-diagonal corners will be shaded since these are the points of maximal difference. In some exceptional cases when it is difficult to identify the meaningful difference, the whole region could be shaded (Panel B, Figure 6.14).

A familiar special case is the categorization of risks. In some fields, the tradition is to create well-accepted risk thresholds, and subsequently, these thresholds then define the risk groups. For example, in cardiovascular research Cook and co-authors [42] used thresholds of 5%, 10%, and 20%. However, for your project, the appropriate thresholds will likely be different and be obtained by a discussion with a subject matter expert. In Panels C and D of Figure 6.14 we have additional examples where the subject matter expert has essentially formed risk groups. Note that if these were risk groups, then the corners of the shaded regions would touch the 45-degree line, such as they do with reclassification. This illustrates the advantage of using the method shown in Panel A of Figure 6.14 over reclassification (Panel D of Figure 6.14) where risks are grouped based on predefined thresholds. With reclassification there are points considered reclassified that are actually closer to the 45-degree line than are points not considered reclassified.

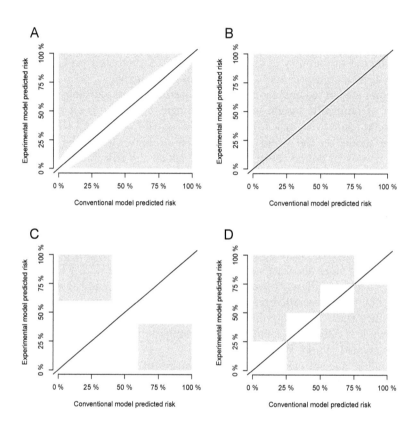

FIGURE 6.14

Examples of clinically relevant changes in prediction. The shaded areas represent differences between conventional and experimental prediction models that have clinical significance. Areas that are not shaded are judged as not clinically different (i.e., of no real practical consequence). If there are many patients in shaded areas, this suggests the more accurately predicting model will also have clinical impact.

6.4 Does a new marker improve prediction?

Before examining a new predictor it is important to recognize the existing predictors. These existing predictors should first be assembled in a model that serves as the benchmark for the upcoming analysis (very much in the same way as we constructed the *conventional model* in Section 6.2). It is quite possible that this has been done already and can be retrieved from the literature. The analyst can still choose to fit his own model rather than using the one from the literature, but doing so necessitates the demonstration of improvement over the existing model from the literature. Consistent with our previous terminology we refer to this benchmark model as the conventional model.

The new model, which we have called the experimental model, contains the new predictor plus predictors from the benchmark model. In a standard regression context, the most direct test of the value of the new predictor is to add its effect to the linear predictor of the conventional model. However, it is not satisfactory to simply conclude that the new marker is helpful based on only its p-value, hazard ratio or odds ratio in the experimental model (Section 2.7.2). It is necessary that the model which contains the new predictor improves prediction performance over the conventional model. To assess this, we compute the change in the Brier score as well as the change in the AUC in a validation dataset in the same way as in Section 6.2. While the statistical community has raised concerns about the validity of Δ AUC [53], this concern is only applicable to settings where the same data are used to train the nested models and to evaluate their Δ AUC [37]. This issue does not apply in our case since an independent test dataset is used for calculating Δ AUC. Thus, meaningful improvement in predictive performance can be assessed by considering the model with the new marker and the conventional model without the new marker as rivals. We now illustrate this by considering two examples. In the oral cancer study, we add the variable tumor grade to the random survival forest model of Section 6.2.2.

```
# R-code
set.seed(1972)
fit1 <- rfsrc(Surv(survtime,survstatus)~ age+tumorthickness+gender+
    tobacco+deep.invasion+site+race+x.posnodes+tumormaxdimension+
    vascular.invasion,data=octrain.cc)
set.seed(1972)
fit2 <- rfsrc(Surv(survtime,survstatus)~ age+tumorthickness+gender+
    tobacco+deep.invasion+site+race+x.posnodes+tumormaxdimension+
    vascular.invasion+Grade,data=octrain.cc)
x <- Score(list("Conventional"=fit1,"New marker"=fit2),
        data=octest.cc,
        formula=Surv(survtime,survstatus)~1,
        times=60,
```

```
            summary=c("risks","IPA"))
plotRisk(x,times=60,preclipse.shade=1,legend.ncol=3,legend.x=0,
    legend.y=1.1,legend.xpd=NA)
mtext("Predicted risk of 5-year mortality",line=2)
```

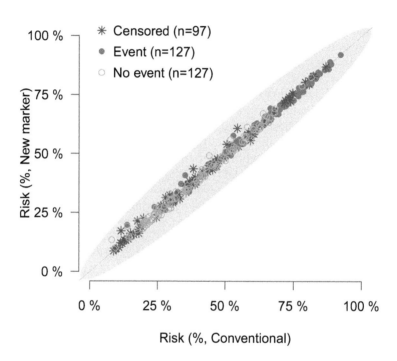

FIGURE 6.15
Oral cancer study. Scatterplot showing test set predictions of 5-year overall survival from a random survival forest model which adds grade versus a conventional random survival forest model. The shaded region indicates the area of clinically meaningless risk difference.

Figure 6.15 demonstrates negligible impact upon predicted probabilities for plot of clinically significant difference shown. This is an extreme case where almost no single person's predicted risk is changed enough to be clinically meaningful. Given this result and the clinically insignificant area, the analysis concludes with no benefit from adding grade to the benchmark. Only for completeness we consider the results of a formal analysis (disregarding the clinically interesting area) that shows that *grade* improves the prediction performance but not significantly (Tables 6.9 and 6.10).

TABLE 6.9
Oral cancer study. Effect of a new marker (*grade*) on the prediction performance of a random survival forest model.

Years	Model	AUC (%)	Brier (%)	IPA
5	Null model	50.0	24.8 [20.3;29.2]	0.0
5	Conventional	77.4 [70.6;84.1]	19.5 [15.4;23.7]	21.2
5	New marker	78.0 [71.2;84.7]	19.3 [15.2;23.4]	22.0

TABLE 6.10
Oral cancer study test set results. Shown is the effect of adding a new predictor variable (grade) to the random survival forest model at the 5-year prediction time horizon.

Years	Model	Ref.	Δ AUC (%)	p-value	Δ Brier (%)	p-value
5	New	Conv.	0.60 [-0.36;1.57]	0.218	-0.21 [-0.61;0.20]	0.314

In the prostate cancer dataset, we assess the effect of adding the ERG status [21] to a prediction model which predicts the 3-year risks of cancer progression based on cause-specific Cox regression models. We use the model from Section 6.2.3 and construct another cause-specific Cox regression model which adds effects of the ERG status on the hazard rate of cancer progression and on the hazard rate of death unrelated to cancer. The scatter plot (Figure 6.16) shows many test set patients outside the clinically insignificant difference region.

```
# R-code
fit1 <- CSC(list(Hist(asprogtime,asprog)~age+psa+ct1+diaggs+ppb5,
    Hist(asprogtime,asprog)~age),data=astrain,cause="progression")
fit2 <- CSC(list(Hist(asprogtime,asprog)~age+psa+ct1+diaggs+ppb5+
    erg.status,Hist(asprogtime,asprog)~age+erg.status),data=
    astrain,cause="progression")
x <- Score(list("Conventional"=fit1,"New marker"=fit2),formula=Hist
    (asprogtime,asprog)~1,cause="progression",data=astest,times=3,
    summary="risks")
plotRisk(x,times=3,xlim=c(0,1),ylim=c(0,1),preclipse.shade=1,legend
    .ncol=3,legend.x=0,legend.y=1,legend.xpd=NA)
mtext("Risk of progression within 3-years",side=3,line=2.3)
```

Test set analysis (disregarding the plot of clinically significant difference) shows that ERG status improves the prediction performance but not significantly (Tables 6.11 and 6.12).

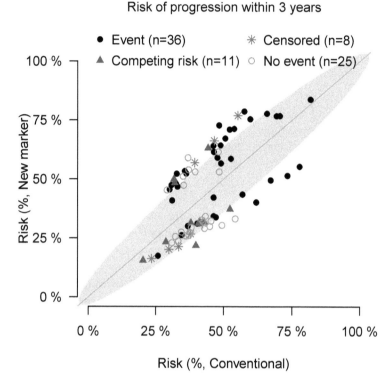

FIGURE 6.16
Active surveillance prostate cancer study. Scatterplot of test set predicted
probabilities from the conventional cause-specific Cox regression model without and with a new marker (ERG status). The shaded region indicates the
area of clinically meaningless risk difference.

TABLE 6.11
Active surveillance prostate cancer study. Test set results. Prediction performance at 3-year prediction time horizon of cause-specific Cox regression with
and without the new marker (ERG status).

Years	Model	AUC (%)	Brier (%)
3	Null model	50.0	24.9 [23.2;26.6]
3	Conventional	70.7 [58.1;83.4]	21.2 [18.4;24.1]
3	New marker	80.4 [70.4;90.4]	18.7 [15.4;22.1]

TABLE 6.12
Active surveillance prostate cancer study test set results. Shown are differences obtained by adding a new predictor variable (ERG status) to a cause-specific Cox regression model as Δ AUC and Δ Brier score at the 3-year prediction time horizon.

Years	Model	Ref.	Δ AUC (%)	p-value	Δ Brier (%)	p-value
3	Exp.	Conv.	9.7 [-2.6;21.9]	0.121	-2.5 [-5.4;0.4]	0.0909

6.4.1 Many new predictors

When searching across many new predictors, the analysis is prone to a multiple testing problem. This is a well-known problem in the analysis of genetic data but can happen in any setting where more than one predictor is examined. The concern here is always that simply by chance a predictor appears to be beneficial, only to find that in a future analysis, the predictor is not. An in-depth discussion of this subject is beyond the scope of our book, but in Chapter 8 we discuss methods for building models that are able to include many predictor variables in one model.

6.4.2 Updating a subject's prediction

There are two settings where updating a subject's prediction commonly occurs. One is where the subject remains free of the event during follow-up and would like a revised estimate of his prediction. No new information is available about him other than he has remained event-free. The statistical term for this form of updating is conditional survival. Say, the subject is requesting his revised prediction after 12 months of follow-up for a prediction horizon of 60 months from the time origin. His revised prediction is simply his original risk divided by the 12-month risk.

In the second setting, additional information is available at the time when the revised prediction is requested. For example, this might be a new blood test result. The statistical terms for this type of updating are dynamic risk prediction and landmark analysis [178, 49, 177]. The date upon which the subject is requesting the revised prediction is called the landmark time point. With this form of updating, the model may actually be refitted by sliding the time origin out to the landmark time point. Only those subjects from the dataset that are alive and event-free at the landmark time point enter the refit analysis. In this setting, one can use short-term outcome information to predict long-term survival [136]. There are also more sophisticated modeling approaches based on joint models [27], models with time-varying coefficients [137, 189], and also R^2-type measures (we call them IPAs) to assess prediction performance across landmark time points [45, 68].

7

What would make me an expert?

In this chapter, we deal with advanced topics that the expert needs to understand and figure out. They arise routinely in the prediction modeling process and require special attention. Many of these issues have no clear solutions but they are still important to recognize. However, even unsolved, these issues are important to point out when discussing the limitations of a study, and potentially could motivate the target of a sensitivity analysis.

7.1 Multiple cohorts / Multi-center studies

Often the researcher receives data from multiple cohorts. These cohorts may come from different hospitals, different doctors, or different countries, as examples. We have to decide whether to simply pool these data or to model them separately. If we pool the data and ignore the source we are assuming there is no difference that persists across cohorts, and the model will perform equally well across cohorts. However, doctors or hospitals or countries will often differ with respect to

- the types of patients that they treat,

- the types of treatment that they use,

- the way they measure predictor variables, and

- the way they measure and monitor outcome (differences in follow-up time).

It is critical to determine whether these differences among cohorts need to be addressed. The concern is that predictions would be meaningfully different, or substantially incorrect, across cohorts. Our examination of the impacts of cohort differences on prediction is analogous to those on marker assessment, described by Meisner et al. [131].

Assume here we presently have all the predictors identified by the subject matter expert in the model. An important first step is to cross-validate by cohort, leaving each one as a holdout while modeling the others. This way we see model performance for each cohort when it alone is used as a test set. If we are lucky, each cohort as a test set shows good predictive accuracy, with consistent discrimination results and only small departures from perfect calibration. How "small" is "small" is a subject matter expert judgment call, but one would like to see that the IPA values do not vary much.

One way to think about this is whether the performance in any holdout sample would be acceptable if it were the only validation dataset. This assessment is much easier in the presence of a rival model or other prediction approach – where one can just judge the new model versus the old one. In that case, hopefully the new model beats the old one in all centers when each is held out. However, perhaps a single small cohort is the culprit, and dropping it from the dataset solves all the problems – the difference among the cohorts goes away. If this is a workable solution, simply leave the pooled data as the modeling dataset; fit the full model; bootstrap the full model; and cross validate by center. Then, all the data are being used for model building and evaluation (the full model and the bootstrapped validation results), and the cohort issue has been removed.

However, if the cohort difference is more complicated than simply solving it by removing a small cohort, the answer is not simple. Recalibration by center is not a good solution since this would imply that predictions at centers outside those used in the analysis would need unknown calibration adjustment before the model could be used. At the extreme, bad calibration across all cohorts argues each center needs to make its own prediction model, and the value of a published, publicly available, prediction tool is small since no one can use it without recalibration or rebuilding. Thus, with clinically meaningful differences across cohorts, there may be no easy solution. Treating the variable as a fixed effect, and simply including it as a covariate, causes a problem for predictions in patients not from those cohorts – the risk calculator would only have values for new patients from one of the "centers" that contributed data to the learning dataset. Thus, this solution should be avoided if the aim is to generalize the model and apply it to patients in centers other than those of the learning dataset.

Including the cohort variable as a random effect in a logistic or Cox regression model would make it possible to predict new patients from other centers. However, doing this is not well motivated. There are two problems. The first is that adding a random effect corresponds to conditioning on another predictor variable (the random effect), although this variable has not been observed. Hence, if the random effect turns out to be important this means that an important predictor variable is not available and hence the predicted risk may be systematically too low or too high. The second problem is related to the non-collapsibility of logistic regression models and Cox regression models [83]. Omitting an important predictor variable (the random effect) leads to attenuation of the estimated regression coefficients toward zero [91, 90]. However, this shrinkage effect is good for prediction as is well known from ridge regression (Section 8.2.1). Hence, including a random effect has the opposite effect of shrinkage and would often decrease the predictive performance. Whatever problems were observed with discrimination, calibration, etc., will remain or will get worse when a random effect is introduced. Ideally, a subject matter expert would explain what is different across the cohorts, as defined by variables not presently included in the model, and those variables could be added to the model. However, typically, the subject matter expert does not really know what is different, or those variables are not measured or available.

Another issue that arises with multi-center studies is that the maximum length of follow-up will differ, at least to an extent. This becomes a particular issue when the prediction horizon exceeds the maximum length of follow-up for one or more of the centers. The prediction model will have to make the untestable assumption that patients in the longer follow-up center(s) are representative of those in shorter follow-up center(s).

Many studies have, of course, simply pooled their data and not followed our recommendation here – there was no cross-validation by center to examine for cohort effects. Perhaps the reason for this was that the researchers did not want to know the answer to this question given how difficult the fix is. But one would have to question the robustness of a model that has never been evaluated in a truly new cohort. However, finding that a model that does well when cross validated across centers speaks to its potential usefulness in settings even beyond the cohorts evaluated, which is the goal for any prediction model.

Another approach that could be used in the presence of a difference across cohorts is to resort to a points-based system. A simple score that puts patients into a handful of groups, depending upon the sum of the score, is more likely to be transportable across the centers. The reason for this transportability is that only discrimination is assessed: Do patients with more points have a worse outcome than those with fewer points? That is, a lower threshold than is typical with statistical prediction models, where calibration is of concern. The other drawback with a points system is that it is crude, and heterogeneity persists for patients with the same number of points. It is easy to have a patient with 3 points to be at higher risk than a patient with 4 points, for example, because the assessment just looks at the group with 3 points versus the group with 4 points. For this reason, a statistical prediction model is generally preferred to a crude and simple points system.

7.2   The role of treatment for making a prediction model

Treatment is different from other risk factors because it can be intervened upon. Indeed, a common task for medical risk prediction models is to help the patient to decide which treatment, if any, to select. A major challenge in this regard is interference with the old or current treatment guidelines: Purpose data collected to build a new risk prediction model are collected in a period where the decision about treatment is influenced by other guidelines or perhaps based on the risk prediction by a *conventional model*.

Unfortunately, there does not seem to be much theoretical or practical guidance in the statistical literature regarding how one should deal with this problem. Simply ignoring the interference with previous guidelines may not be the best solution for modeling. When only one treatment has been modeled, it is easiest to say that the model is not to be used for selecting a treatment but to be used after the treatment has been selected to verify that the treatment choice is a good one. As an example, consider a model that predicts failure after surgery. In the purpose dataset, all patients received surgery. Therefore, the model may not be helpful for convincing patients who were not a good fit for surgery previously to now have surgery since, theoretically, they would not be in the purpose dataset. Instead, the model is used to make sure the patient still wants surgery after the failure risk has been predicted. Furthermore, a similar problem occurs in the form of feedback when a newly developed model is validated in future patients who are treated according to a new protocol which involves the risk prediction of the new model regarding treatment decision. It is important to attempt to restrict the analysis to patients who would theoretically fit both the conventional and new prediction model.

7.2.1 Modeling treatment

Suppose within the cohort (and thus within the purpose dataset) some patients received treatment while others did not. The first issue to clarify is whether the treatment here, which is directly related to the outcome event of interest, i.e., a treatment for which the decision about initiation should, in the future, be based on the medical prediction model that we are about to make. (All other treatments can be considered risk factors and can be used to characterize the patients at the time origin and/or to define the target population.)

For example, the aim of the CHA_2DS_2VASC score [71] is to guide patients with artrial fibrillation whether or not to initiate blood thinning (anticoagulation) therapy to prevent stroke. Suppose the aim is to build a new medical prediction model for atrial fibrillation patients which aims to provide improved risk predictions compared to the CHA_2DS_2VASC score. Then, an issue that the modeler needs to deal with is that some patients in the purpose dataset received anticoagulation therapy, and likely the decision was guided by the CHA_2DS_2VASC score. What options are there for the modeler? Using anticoagulation therapy (at the time origin) as one of the predictor variables to predict the outcome risk is tricky because the new model would implicitly assume that the conventional model, i.e., the CHA_2DS_2VASC score, is initially used to decide about treatment. Similarly, a subgroup analysis of treated and untreated would implicitly depend on the propensity of treatment in the purpose dataset (which was guided by the CHA_2DS_2VASC score).

Anyway, often we would like to provide risk predictions with and without treatment, more generally with all possible treatment options (see Section 7.2.2), and thereby help the patient to make the decision. One potential solution for the modeling is to simply separate the purpose datasets by treatment and then repeat all steps of modeling (Chapter 4) and validation (Chapters 5 and 6). This would lead to treatment-specific risk prediction models. If treatment was randomly assigned at the time origin and if a sufficient amount of data is available for all treatment options, then this could potentially be a straightforward analysis. However, in many settings, the treatment decision was not randomized for the patients in the cohort behind the purpose dataset, or there were treatment drop-ins that the modeler would like to account for [164]. One problem that might arise is that the treated look different from the untreated patients, i.e., in terms of their predictor variables. This would naturally be the case when the treatment initiation depended on the predictor variables because a conventional risk prediction model was applied or due to other guidelines and habits. In order to address this situation, the modeler needs to enter the realm of causal inference [96] and discuss *positivity* and *exchangeability*.

To explain *positivity*, suppose the treated patients (who contribute to the purpose dataset) are all under age 50 while the untreated patients are all over 40. Going forward the prediction of the outcome probability assuming treatment will not be available for patients over 50. Any attempt to correct this would require extrapolation beyond the limits of observed data, because there are no data of patients older than 50 who received the treatment (violation of the positivity assumption).

To explain *exchangeability*, suppose that the patients whose data are available for modeling were not randomized to treatment. In simple regression analysis, this could make treatment always look like the better option even if it has no effect. To be able to correct for this bias, one would need to try to translate between the observed world (where treatment was not randomized) and a hypothetical world in which treatment was randomized. In the hypothetical world, each patient has a clone who is receiving the treatment if the patient in the real world was untreated. Likewise, the clone in the hypothetical world is untreated if the patient in the real world received treatment. If there are unmeasured confounders, i.e., variables associated with both the treatment assignment and the outcome, but these are not observed, then it may be not possible to achieve an unbiased interpretation of the predicted risk under all treatment options (violation of the exchangeability assumption). In addition to the positivity and exchangeability assumptions, one further needs to worry about the *consistency* assumption. *Consistency* requires that there is only one way to administer the treatment, and it does not matter whether the patient is randomized to the treatment or whether treatment is a consequence of guidelines, advice from a doctor, or personal preference.

Using tools from causal inference, it is potentially possible to build models that predict the risks of the event for a new patient under multiple alternative treatment plans.

7.2.2 Comparative effectiveness tables

Comparative effectiveness involves the comparison of treatment strategies, side by side, with respect to expected outcomes [175]. These outcomes are typically benefits and harms, expressed as probabilities (chances of benefit and risks of harm). In that way, a meaningful comparison can be made of the treatment choices under consideration. Say, for example, there are two treatments available, and one benefit and one harm is each at stake. For example, consider a patient who is newly diagnosed with atrial fibrillation and needs to start anticoagulation therapy. The decision between two anticoagulation drugs is guided by the benefit of a lower risk of stroke and the harmful effect of an increased risk of bleeding. We would build four statistical prediction models: one for each outcome/treatment combination. Those predictions would be placed side by side in a 2x2 *comparative effectiveness table* to provide risk predictions for future patients. It is not different if there are more than two outcomes or more than two treatments: one makes a statistical prediction model for each treatment/outcome combination. However, one needs to address whether one outcome is a competing risk for another outcome (Sections 2.1.3 and 2.4.6). Also, one needs a sufficient amount of data from previous patients for each treatment option, and one needs to worry about *positivity, exchangeability* and *consistency* (Section 7.2.1).

An important concern with comparative effectiveness tables is residual confounding (*exchangeability*). Unless the data underlying the models come from randomized controlled trials of the treatments being featured in the comparative effectiveness tables, one has to worry about whether the prediction models properly adjust for all important covariates.

Consider the example of the drug Dutasteride for the prevention of prostate cancer [134]. This drug is controversial because it might lower the risk of prostate cancer in general yet raise the risk of an aggressive prostate cancer subtype. Moreover, the drug has some pleasant side effects as well as some undesirable side effects. Thus, there are tradeoffs with this drug, so it is important that a patient is fully informed of the advantages and disadvantages before taking the drug. But the risks of the good and bad outcomes depend on many things, such as the age of the patient, symptoms, blood test results, and other medical exams.

Note that a comparative effectiveness table generally does not tell an individual patient what to do. Instead, the patient is provided with the most accurate outcome predictions currently available. He or she must then consider his or her own preferences for those outcomes, and how strongly he or she feels about avoiding or experiencing them. For the Dutasteride decision making there are 9 different outcomes to consider (cancer risks, side effects, etc.). The choice comes down to two options: take the drug or do not. Thus, our comparative effectiveness table, in the form of a risk calculator, comes down to a 2 by 9 grid of options versus outcomes. We place the predictor vari-

ables and the outcomes on a single screen so that the comparative effectiveness
table is easily updated as the inputs vary (Figure 7.1)

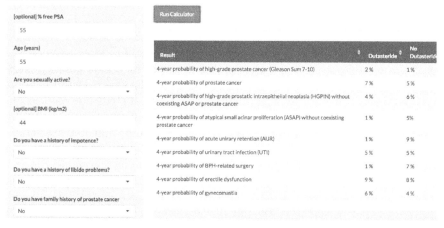

Patients at High Risk for Prostate Cancer - with a Prior Negative 6- to 12-Core Biopsy in
the Past 6 Months

FIGURE 7.1
Example of a comparative effectiveness table with two treatment options:
Dutasteride and no Dutasteride.

7.3   Learning curve paradigm

This section describes the learning curve paradigm, which is not at all a surprising assumption but important to keep in mind when dealing with internal
validation schemes (Section 7.4) and missing values in the predictor variables
(Section 7.5). Both issues force the modeler to apply the modeling strategy to
subsets of the full purpose dataset.

Learning curve paradigm: We assume that the more data are available for
modeling, i.e., the larger the size of the purpose dataset, the better the risk
prediction model will perform – no matter the modeling strategy.

It thus makes sense to assume that the learning curve of our algorithm
increases as a function of the sample size of the purpose dataset (Figure 7.2).
The dilemma of the modeler who has only one purpose dataset to build and
validate the model is that, even though interest is in the conditional performance of the model built with all data, none of the estimates described in

Section 7.4 correlates well with it [59] (see also [89]). We discuss this further in Section 7.4.4.

7.4   Internal validation (data splitting)

Theoretically, what we really want to know is how well a statistical prediction model will predict when applied to future patients. Unfortunately, we can never know how well a model will do in future patients; we have to do our best to estimate this because the future patient is always in front of us.

In many applications, the greatest challenge for any attempt to estimate the performance of a model is the lack of data for the purpose. Two typical approaches are widely used: single split and cross-validation. Both have their strengths and weaknesses, so neither can outright be advocated above the other; they should be evaluated individually based on context. Here we discuss each and why they are often used. We use the following synonyms:

- *learning set = training set =* {data used to build the model}

- *validation set = test set =* {data used to evaluate the model}

7.4.1   Single split

The single-split approach hides part of the data from **all steps** of model building and then estimates the *conditional performance* of the final model using the left-out part of the data (Figure 7.3).

A great advantage of this approach is that one does not have to pre-specify the steps of modeling. In fact, with this approach the model-building process is allowed to use the learning set in any way and may combine expert opinion (e.g., regarding which predictor variables should enter the model) with data-dependent decisions (e.g., removing a non-significant predictor variable to simplify the model). The attraction of the single-split approach, which applies to machine learning approaches as well as to standard regression approaches, is that many adjustments and tuning parameters can be adjusted during the training session. Often these adjustments require human judgment or intervention and are difficult to prespecify. The single-split approach lets the modeler do whatever he or she wants on the learning data as long as the testing data are not examined until the final model is locked down.

A major drawback of this approach is the dependence of the results on which part of the data is hidden. Both the risk predictions of the model and the estimate of model performance are affected by how exactly the data are split, i.e., which patients are in the learning set and which patients are in the validation set. When this is done at random, the result will depend on the random seed. With R software this is controlled with the function set.seed.

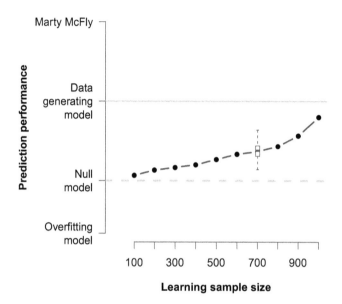

FIGURE 7.2

Illustration of the learning curve paradigm: The prediction performance of
a model is increasing with increasing learning sample size. The points on
the black line represent the average performance across all possible learning
datasets of a given sample size. The boxplot shows the variability of the performance across different learning datasets (all having the same sample size,
here illustrated at n=700). The lower benchmark is obtained with the null
model (see Chapter 4). The upper benchmark is obtained with the "data-
generating model" which assigns the correct probability of the event to each
patient. Only Marty McFly (see the movie, Back to the Future) is able to
travel in time to the prediction horizon to know the outcome at the prediction
horizon and achieve perfect prediction performance by going back in time to
predict either 0% or 100%.

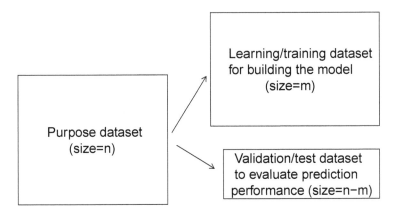

FIGURE 7.3

A single split of the data according to a split ratio m/n requires a choice of m and a way to choose the n-m subjects from the purpose dataset. The data reserved for testing performance may, under no circumstances, be touched during the model-building process. Usually, the data-building process consists not just of the estimation of regression parameters, but includes everything, and in particular the selection of variables. The results of the single-split approach depend on the random seed.

It is not easy to explain what the random seed is in English. But it controls the random number generator, which in turn affects how data are split.

Another important drawback of the single-split approach is that, eventually, part of the purpose dataset is not used to build the final model. When the single-split approach is used to allow the analyst to make modeling decisions by looking at the data, the final model has a performance evaluation that is dependent on the particular split of the data (e.g., a random number seed selected by the analyst), and data were wasted for model development. This model should not be implemented in clinical practice.

For the sole purpose of illustration, we worked out the oral cancer example in Chapter 6.2.2 using a single split of the complete cases (no missing values in any of the predictor variables) of the oral cancer data. The estimate of the difference in Brier scores at the 5-year prediction time horizon for the specific random split used to obtain the learning and validation sets is Δ Brier = -1.05% (Table 6.4). Table 7.1 illustrates that this result depends significantly on the random seed used to split the data into the learning and validation sets.

```
-----------------------pseudo-code---------------------------

Repeat 1-4 for different starting values of
the random number generator(seeds):

1. set seed
2. split data into learning and validation sets
3. fit rival models to learning set
4. use validation set to calculate difference in Brier score

-----------------------pseudo-code---------------------------
```

```r
# R-code
foreach(s=c(9,4991,175)) %do% { # loop the value s through
  # three different start values
  # for the random number generator
  set.seed(s)
  N <- NROW(oc.cc) # total sample size
  M <- round(0.632*NROW(oc.cc)) # learning sample size
  oc.cc$inbag <- 1:N%in%sample(1:N,replace=FALSE,size=M) # random
    split variable (TRUE for learning, FALSE for validation)
  train <- oc.cc[inbag==TRUE,]
  test <- oc.cc[inbag==FALSE,]
  # fit models in learning set
  fit1 <- cph(Surv(survtime,survstatus)~rcs(age,3)+tumorthickness+
    gender+tobacco+deep.invasion+site+race+x.posnodes+
    tumormaxdimension+vascular.invasion,
        data=train, x=TRUE, y=TRUE, surv=TRUE)
  # seed for random forest
  set.seed(1972)
  fit2 <- rfsrc(Surv(survtime,survstatus)~ age+tumorthickness+
    gender+tobacco+deep.invasion+site+race+x.posnodes+
    tumormaxdimension+vascular.invasion,data=train)
  x <- Score(list("Conventional"=fit1, # trained Cox regression
        "Experimental"=fit2), # trained Random forest
      data=test, # test set
      formula=Surv(survtime,survstatus)~1,
      times=60, # prediction time horizon
      )$Brier$contrast[3]$delta # difference in Brier score
}
```

However, even before considering the effect on the performance metric of how the data are split into learning and validation sets, one should be aware of the effect on the individualized predicted risks. Figure 7.4 shows random seed effects on individual predicted risks for three example patients of the oral cancer study and varying learning sample size. To obtain the data shown by the boxplots in Figure 7.4, the following three steps were repeated 100 times for each learning sub-sample size V:

TABLE 7.1

Oral cancer study. Δ Brier is the difference in prediction performance between the Cox regression and the random survival forest model (c.f., Table 6.4). Shown is the effect of the random seed (three different starting values for the random number generator) used to split the data into a learning set and a validation set.

seed	Δ Brier
9	-1.3
4991	-0.4
175	-2.7

1. A learning dataset including V patients is drawn without replacement from the oral cancer dataset.

2. The Cox regression model of Section 6.2.2 is fitted to the learning data.

3. The resulting model is used to predict the 5-year risk of all-cause mortality in three example patients with a low, medium and high risk profile, respectively.

For a given sample size n, the split ratio defines an integer $m < n$ such that the data of m subjects are used for building the model and the data of the remaining $n - m$ subjects are reserved for estimating model performance. When a single dataset is split into training and testing, it can be split into 50% for training and 50% testing, or 75/25, or 80/20, or any potential split. A commonly used choice is what we could call the *golden split of statistics*, which defines m such that the learning set contains 63.2% of the purpose data; note that the probability to draw (with replacement) any specific subject from a dataset of any given size is 63.2% (see also corresponding R-code in Section 7.4.3).

For example, when the total sample size is $n = 733$, as in the complete case scenario of our oral cancer study, then, following this split ratio, one would split the data into a learning set of size $m = 463$ and use the remaining $n - m = 270$ subjects to estimate the performance of the model built on the learning data. However, there seem to be no theoretical arguments and no generally applicable practical arguments for this particular choice, or any other choice for the value of the split ratio. Hence, there is no good reason to favor one over another single-split ratio value; one is trading the quantity of data available for training versus the quantity available for testing the model. Clearly there is a tradeoff: the more data we use for training the model, the better the prediction model will perform, and the more data we use for testing the performance, the closer the estimate of performance will be to the true unknown performance of the model.

Unfortunately, the single-split approach might allow the modeler to get

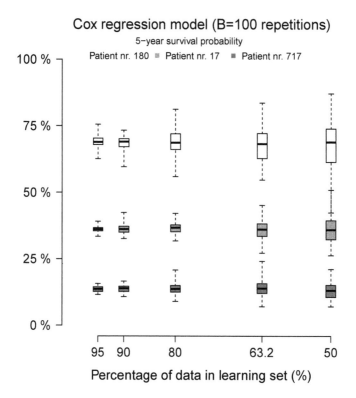

FIGURE 7.4

The variation of individualized predicted risks obtained from 100 models trained in 100 learning datasets obtained by drawing patients at random from the complete cases (no missing values in the predictor variables) of the oral cancer study. A popular choice is 10-fold cross-validation where 90% of the data are in the learning set. The variability of the predictions of three example patients increases with increasing split ratio, i.e., decreasing size of the learning set.

lucky with whatever was done because there is only one test set examined, and with a different random seed the results could change significantly (see Table 7.1). This can be abused if the modeler tries different things, each with a different random seed (to control how the data are split), and then reports the session where the test set performance is best. Such trial and error with selective reporting is highly biased and not at all representative of what to expect in future patients. In other words, we need to trust that investigators are not trying several different random seeds to modify the results in accordance with other scientific or non-scientific claims.

Another concern is that the analyst might split the data and try something that does not predict well. He or she changes something (e.g., a tuning parameter), splits the data once, and checks again. He or she might repeat this process many times and stop when a nice result is found. This is biased if only the last setting is reported. We have pointed out the many drawbacks of a single split, urging the modeler to do multiple splits. We realize this may be daunting since all steps of the modeling process (e.g., variable selection, category merging, continuous variable transformation) need to be including in each repetition of the split process (modeling and testing), and that level of programming may be out of reach. If so, a single split may be the only practical option. Although the single split has many drawbacks, it is still better than no split at all.

We should note that all the real data illustrations of Chapters 5 and 6 are obtained with a single-split approach which depends on the specific seed for the random number generator. However, in those chapters the aim was solely to illustrate the methods. If the model that results from the single-split approach was to be implemented in clinical practice and applied to new patients, the drawbacks of this approach may become a real problem when, as is usually the case, the results are highly sensitive to how the data were split. A reviewer of such a model could argue that the predicted risks are random numbers (they depend on the random seed selected by the investigators) and suboptimal because a model which one could build in all data would likely outperform the current model.

Below we discuss two alternative approaches (calendar split and cross-validation); both achieve two common aims: We get rid of the randomness of the results and we use the full purpose dataset (not a smaller learning set) to build the best possible model. Both approaches require that a recipe for the model-building process has been pre-specified with all its data-dependent steps. In addition, for cross-validation we need a computer program that implements the model-building process.

7.4.2 Calendar split

An interesting alternative to a single random split becomes available when the subjects, whose data are in the purpose dataset, were enrolled over time. In this case, a natural estimate of the prediction performance in future patients is obtained by hiding the data of the subjects enrolled in the latest calendar period. The latest calendar period could, for example, be the last year of the enrollment period. It may be possible to process along a sequence of calendar time periods, e.g., years, by building model-x with data up to the calendar year x and to estimate the performance of model-x with the data of subjects enrolled after x. A feature of such a sequence of model building and model testing is that the size of the learning sets increases, whereas the size of the validation sets decreases. A limitation may be that the probability of being censored at the prediction horizon may be relatively high in validation sets consisting of the latest subjects. Also, if calendar time is one of the predictors used in the modeling, then special attention has to be paid because the risks in future patients are obtained by extrapolation.

Based on this approach, if the recipe for building the model can be specified such that computer code can produce the model, then the same computer code can be applied at the very end to the full dataset including all years up to year y. In this way, one obtains a model that can be applied to future patients. Under the assumption that the prediction performance of the model is not decreasing with increasing calendar time, the performance of model-y can be approximated by the performance of model-(y-1). Since the size of the learning set increases, this seems generally a reasonable assumption, unless indicated differently in a specific subject matter situation.

7.4.3   Multiple splits (cross-validation)

The multi-split approach repeats the single-split approach many times and averages the performance results across the splits. This requires that all data-dependent steps of modeling are available in the form of an algorithm (computer program). The parameters of the multi-split approach are as follows:

1. How the learning data are obtained from the purpose data. Common options are k-fold cross-validation, regular bootstrap, and subsample bootstrap.

2. The number of times the data are split, i.e., how many times the algorithm is applied. For example, when 10-fold cross-validation is repeated 5 times then there are 50 learning sets and 50 test sets.

3. The split ratio defines the relative size of the learning datasets. See Figure 7.5.

4. How the performance is averaged across the test sets.

It is important to note that the multi-split approach is most useful to compare rival modeling algorithms and does not directly address the conditional performance of the particular model obtained with one of the modeling algorithms in the full purpose dataset. Rather, we estimate the average performance of the algorithms across learning sets (see Figure 7.2). In each split of the process of any cross-validation scheme, the algorithm is applied to the

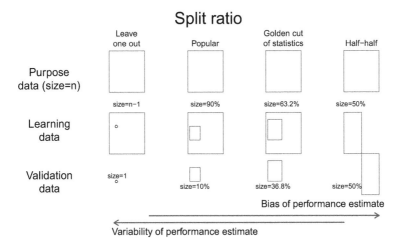

FIGURE 7.5
The split ratio determines how many different individuals are in the learning
and validation datasets, respectively, in each step of the cross-validation algorithm. How exactly depends on the actual cross-validation scheme/algorithm.

learning dataset to build a prediction model (see Figure 2.5). By design, the
training data contain less information than the full purpose dataset, and this
affects the interpretation of the average performance.

> *As soon as we have identified the best-performing modeling algorithm
> via cross-validation, the algorithm is applied once more to build the final
> model using the full purpose dataset.*

However, in many situations it makes sense to believe that the algorithm
which performs best on average will also yield the best prediction model when
it is applied to any particular dataset. Under this assumption, a good way to
exploit the full purpose dataset is to first apply multi-split cross-validation to
select the best algorithm and then obtain the final model by applying it to
the full purpose dataset.

The multi-split approach is nice because it removes the possibility that
some single random split of the data resulted in better than expected performance. It usually requires many splits to achieve a result that is sufficiently
independent of the random seed. By this we could, for example, mean that
the variation of the random seed affects only the 4th decimal of the results,
i.e., such that the changes in the Brier score and AUC do not matter.

A popular scheme is 10-fold cross-validation. First, the purpose dataset is
split at random into 10 approximately equally sized subsets. Second, the first

subset is removed and the rival modeling algorithms are applied to build rival prediction models using the remaining 90% of the purpose dataset. Third, the resulting rival prediction models are applied to predict the outcome of the patients in the first subset. Fourth, the second and third steps are repeated for all other subsets and in this way predicted risks are collected for each patient in the purpose dataset (using prediction models which were trained without this patient). Fifth, the prediction performance (Brier score, AUC) is calculated by comparing the predicted risks with the actual outcome of the patients. Figure 7.6 illustrates this procedure for 3-fold cross-validation.

Unfortunately, the result of 10-fold cross-validation applied once is often still random in the sense that when we repeat it using a different (random) split of the data in 10 equally large pieces, the results change considerably. To improve this, one can repeat 10-fold cross-validation many times, for example 40 times, and then average the 40 estimates of performance. In this case, one would have to apply the modeling algorithm 400 times (10 times in each of 40 repetitions of 10-fold cross-validation). Alternatively, one could average 100 repetitions of 4-fold cross-validation also building 400 models. However, with 4-fold the learning sets are smaller compared with 10-fold cross-validation. There seems to be no generally applicable rule to choose the value k of k-fold cross-validation, but more repetition is certainly better. In order to know when one can safely stop repeating k-fold one would need a convergence criterion based on the Monte-Carlo error.

To illustrate 10-fold cross-validation we consider the situation in Section 6.2.2 and compare the conventional model (Cox regression) with the experimental model (random survival forest) in the data of the oral cancer study.

```
# R-code (takes a while to run, use multiple cores to speed up)
fit1 <- cph(Surv(survtime,survstatus)~rcs(age,3)+tumorthickness+
    gender+tobacco+deep.invasion+site+race+x.posnodes+
    tumormaxdimension+vascular.invasion,
        data=oc.cc, x=TRUE, y=TRUE, surv=TRUE)
set.seed(1972)
fit2 <- rfsrc(Surv(survtime,survstatus)~ age+tumorthickness+gender+
    tobacco+deep.invasion+site+race+x.posnodes+tumormaxdimension+
    vascular.invasion,data=oc.cc)
x <- Score(list("Conventional"=fit1,"Experimental"=fit2),
        data=oc.cc,
        formula=Surv(survtime,survstatus)~1,
        times=60,
        split.method="cv10", # 10-fold cross-validation
        B=10, # repeat 10-fold 10 times
        seed=9, # fix randomness of the splits
        se.fit=0, # no standard errors
        ncpus=2,  # number of cores on computer
        summary="IPA")
summary(x,what="score")[[1]]
```

Compared to the single-split results (see Table 6.3), the cross-validation

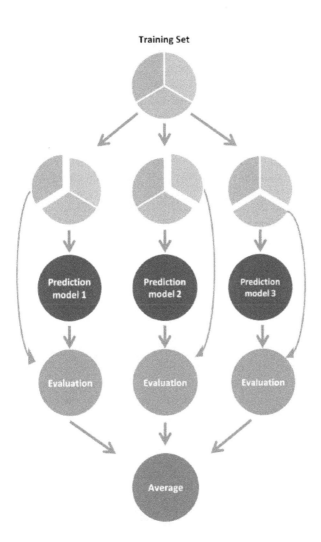

FIGURE 7.6
Illustration of 3-fold cross-validation.

TABLE 7.2

Results of repeating 10-fold cross-validation 10 times for the conventional model (Cox regression) and the experimental model (random survival forest) using the complete case data (no missing predictor variables) of the oral cancer study at the 5-year prediction time horizon.

times	Model	AUC (%)	Brier (%)	IPA
60	Null model	50.0	24.9	0.0
60	Conventional	74.6	20.0	19.7
60	Experimental	75.8	19.2	22.7

performance of the conventional model is higher (both higher AUC and lower Brier). For the experimental model the cross-validated Brier score is lower and the cross-validated AUC is also lower. However, the interpretation of the conditional performance results in Table 6.3 and the average performance results in Table 7.2 are not the same (see Figure 7.2) and hence it is not too useful to compare the two tables. Anyway, we may conclude that the particular single split used to illustrate the methods in Chapter 6 was in favor of the experimental model.

The bootstrap for evaluation of prediction models, as developed by Efron [57, 59], is an alternative to k-fold cross-validation. Here we need to distinguish the regular bootstrap from the subsampling bootstrap. Both are methods to split the purpose dataset into learning and validation sets. The regular bootstrap defines learning datasets by drawing with replacement from the purpose dataset so that the size of each learning dataset is equal to the size of the purpose dataset. In this way, we expect that 63.2% different subjects contribute with one or several lines of data to a learning dataset. The reason for this is that the probability of drawing a single subject, with replacement, is 63.2%, regardless of the sample size. In the following code, the subject number (here 8) and the sample size (here n=399) can be changed without changing the results (up to Monte-Carlo error). The result is an approximation of the probability based on B=10,000 simulations.

```
# R-code
set.seed(71)
B=10000
subject=8
sample.size=399
mean(sapply(1:B,function(b){
    subject%in%sample(1:sample.size,replace=TRUE)
}))
```

```
[1] 0.6319
```

It then follows that if we sample with replacement until we have as many subjects (with repetition) in the bootstrap sample as in the original dataset, the bootstrap set will contain data from approximately 63.2% unique subjects. When the sample size is 399 we expect ≈ 252 unique subjects:

```
# R-code
set.seed(71)
B=10000
sample.size=399
mean(sapply(1:B,function(b){
    length(unique(sample(1:sample.size,replace=TRUE)))
}))
```

[1] 252.4034

The subjects who are not drawn into the bootstrap set compose the test set. Thus, with regular bootstrap the average size of the test sets is 36.8%. The subsampling bootstrap, on the other hand, defines the learning datasets by drawing *without* replacement according to a given split-ratio. For example, if the split-ratio is 80:20, then in each split we draw 80% of (unique) patients into the learning dataset and use the remaining 20% as the validation set.

When the multiple-split approach uses the bootstrap (regular or subsampling) to draw learning sets, then there are two alternative ways to average the results across the splits. The first is intuitive: calculate the performance (Brier score, AUC) in each test set and then average the performances across test sets. The result is called the *bootstrap cross-validation* estimate of prediction performance [132]. To illustrate the *bootstrap cross-validation* estimate of prediction performance we consider again the setting of Section 6.4.

```
# R-code
fit1 <- CSC(list(Hist(asprogtime,asprog)~age+psa+ct1+diaggs+ppb5,
    Hist(asprogtime,asprog)~age),data=astrain,cause="progression")
fit2 <- CSC(list(Hist(asprogtime,asprog)~age+psa+ct1+diaggs+ppb5+
    erg.status,Hist(asprogtime,asprog)~age+erg.status),data=
    astrain,cause="progression")
x <- Score(list("Conventional"=fit1,"New marker"=fit2),
    formula=Hist(asprogtime,asprog)~1,
    cause="progression",
    seed=7,   # fix randomness of the split
    split.method="bootcv",# bootstrap cross-validation
    B=200, # number of subsample bootstraps
    M=0.632*NROW(as), # learning sample size
    data=as,
    times=3,
    summary="risks")
summary(x,what="score")
```

The values shown as [upper;lower] in Table 7.3 are not confidence intervals in the normal statistical sense, but represent the 2.5% and 97.5% quantiles

TABLE 7.3
Active surveillance prostate cancer study. Test set results. Prediction performance at 3-year prediction time horizon of cause-specific Cox regression with and without the new marker (ERG status).

times	Model	AUC (%)	Brier (%)
3	Null model	50.0	25.1 [23.6;27.6]
3	Conventional	62.1 [51.9;72.1]	23.8 [21.0;26.9]
3	New marker	72.3 [63.0;82.6]	21.3 [17.7;25.0]

of the 200 test set results from the 200 splits of the purpose data into learning and test sets. Comparing these results with those of Table 6.11 nicely illustrates the dependence of the single-split approach on the particular random seed. The variability of the results is quite large as shown in Table 7.3.

However, instead of *bootstrap cross-validation*, a better alternative for averaging the results across multiple splits is called *leave-one-out bootstrap* [59]. Here, for each subject in the purpose dataset, one collects the predictions of all those splits where the subject ended up in the test set. These predictions are compared with the outcome of the subjects at the time horizon to form residuals (Brier scores of subject in splits), and the average residual (average Brier score of subject) is calculated for each subject. The *leave-one-out bootstrap* estimate of prediction performance is then the average of the subject-specific average residuals (Brier score of prediction model). Similarly a *leave-two-out bootstrap* is available for the AUC [188].

There are two advantages of the *leave-one-out bootstrap* over *bootstrap cross-validation*. The first is that the form of the *leave-one-out bootstrap* allows one to estimate the standard error of the estimate via the *jackknife after bootstrap* [59, 188]. The second is that for a head-to-head comparison of models (statistical test), the *leave-one-out bootstrap* allows us to directly compare the models' predictions on the same subject very much in the same way as the one-sample (or paired) t-test.

To illustrate the *leave-one-out* bootstrap scheme, we consider the example of Section 6.2.1. The *jackknife after bootstrap* standard errors are used to construct confidence intervals and p-values. In Section 6.2.1 we assessed the test set performance of the conventional and experimental models obtained with a learning sub-sample of the in vitro fertilization study data. Now we assess the performance across conventional and experimental models obtained in 200 regular bootstrap samples.

```
# R-code
fit1 <- lrm(ohss~ant.foll+cyclelen+smoking+age,data=ivftrain)
fit2 <- lrm(ohss~rcs(ant.foll,3)*smoking+cyclelen+age+fsh+bmi+
    ovolume,data=ivftrain,penalty=10)
x <- Score(list("Conventional"=fit1,"Experimental"=fit2),
    data=ivftest, formula=ohss~1,
```

```
    split.method="loob", # leave-one-out bootstrap
    seed=8, # fix randomness of the split
    B=200,  # number of regular bootstrap sets
    summary="ipa")
summary(x,what="contrasts")
```

TABLE 7.4
In vitro fertilization study. Leave-one-out bootstrap results comparing the experimental model (Exp.) with the conventional model (Conv.) in terms of differences of prediction performance. The results are based on fitting the models in 200 regular bootstrap learnings sets (with replacement).

Model	Reference	Δ AUC (%)	p-value	Δ Brier (%)	p-value
Exp.	Conv.	1.5 [-1.8;4.8]	0.3853	-0.8 [-2.7;1.2]	0.4483

Here we see that the experimental model(ing strategy) is not providing much improvement, if any, over the conventional model(ing strategy). The AUC is greater by 0.015, while the Brier is lower by 0.8, though neither of these differences appears significantly different from zero. Still, one would likely switch to the experimental model unless there is a large cost to switch from the conventional or if the conventional model is much faster to execute. Note that we do not care that the improvement in the performance of the experimental model is not statistically significant.

7.4.4 Dilemma of internal validation

The dilemma of internal validation is that the performance parameter in each of the multiple-split approaches via cross-validation is not really the one of interest for the clinical application. We would like to report the performance of the one and only prediction model built with all available data, but we only get to estimate the average performance of the many prediction models that our algorithm builds in multiple learning datasets which are subsets or bootstrap datasets of the purpose data. So, instead of assessing the performance of the model, we assess the performance of the algorithm when we apply the multi-split approach [54]. As soon as the algorithm implements non-smooth data-dependent decisions, such as variable selection, or many regression parameters, the predictions of the model built in any subset or bootstrap set will often deviate considerably from the predictions of the model built with all data. Also, the split-ratio matters, as illustrated in Figure 7.4. Moreover, the sample size will matter in this regard. To this end, note that with regular resampling bootstrap the size of the learning set is the same as the size of the purpose dataset, but the contents of the bootstrap learning datasets are still different and contain less information ($\approx 36.8\%$ less patients) than the purpose dataset.

So, even after we have used the multi-split approach to internal validation, we would usually still want to move forward to clinical practice with the model built with all available purpose data. The performance of this model is then not available (until we have collected new external validation data), but based on the learning curve paradigm (Section 7.3) it would often make sense to assume that the multi-split results are a lower bound for the prediction performance of this model.

7.4.5   The apparent and the .632+ estimator

Because the learning datasets of the multi-split approach always contain less information (data of fewer subjects) compared to the purpose dataset, this implies that the *average performance* estimated by the multi-split approach is systematically lower than the (unknown) *conditional performance* of the model built with all data. The *apparent* or *resubstitution* performance of a prediction model is obtained when the same dataset is used both for building the model and for estimating the performance. It is well known that the performance of the model is overestimated in this way. The general idea of Efron's sequence of estimators for the error rate of a classifier is to average the apparent performance (too high) with the result of a multi-split performance (too low) in a clever way.

The first estimator which improves cross-validation [57] is obtained by training the algorithm in a regular bootstrap dataset and then using all data to estimate the performance. In this way, part of the data ($\approx 36.8\%$) are "new" to the model and part are resubstituted ($\approx 63.2\%$). This method, however, does not work very well for machine learning algorithms.

A more generally applicable approach is the .632 estimator, which linearly combines the apparent performance (with weight .368) and the leave-one-out bootstrap performance (with weight .632). The most sophisticated performance estimator is the .632+ estimator [59], which makes the weights of the .632 dependent on the algorithm by estimating the systematic overfit of the algorithm in perturbed no-information versions of the purpose dataset. Originally proposed for the error rate of a classifier, this method has been adapted for the Brier score [75] and ROC curves [2].

7.4.6   Tips and tricks

1. Number of splits

   Theoretically, we would perform all possible partitions of the dataset for a given split ratio. In most practical settings, however, this requires run times that are too long. To achieve reliable results, the parameter which determines the number of splits should be large enough to make the results robust against human preference – ideally, a convergence criterion and algorithm should control the progress and stop when sufficient precision is reached.

2. Parallelization

   The multi-split approach is perfectly suited for parallel programming because the model-building process in the learning dataset of a particular split is completely independent of the other splits. Thus, if the computational cost of building the model(s) is relatively large, then the total run time can be reduced considerably.

3. Reproducibility

   The performance results should also be reproducible with exact decimals and this requires control of the randomness of the splits which, depending on the system, requires setting the random seed. If parallelization is utilized it may be required to set the random seed explicitly for each worker.

4. Multiple layers of cross-validation and bootstrapping

   When evaluating prediction performance, double and even triple layers of cross-validation and bootstrap occur frequently. For example, when the aim is to assess the prediction performance of a random forest model, then the learning dataset of each split (or fold) will be bootstrapped by the forest algorithm (Section 8.3.1). If the modeling algorithm also tunes some of the random forest's hyperparameters by cross-validation, the number of trees for example, then three layers of cross-validation/bootstrap are at play.

   In such cases, it is important to use subsampling bootstrap and not regular bootstrap for the multi-split approach, i.e., the outermost cross-validation layer. This is to not dilute the intent of the inner cross-validation layer(s). Such misguidance would happen when the outer cross-validation layer draws learning datasets from the purpose data with replacement, because a random split of a regular bootstrap sample will have overlap between training and test datasets, diluting the intention of cross-validation.

5. Tuning

   Any tuning of learning algorithms should focus on the prediction problem and use prediction performance as the criterion function whenever possible. For example, the penalty parameters of an elastic net (Section 8.2.1) could be selected with the Brier score or AUC instead of the default criterion.

6. Individual predictions

   Never forget that the targets of the analysis are the individual predictions. It is too tempting to only look at average performance. However, a model (algorithm) can outperform the rival models (algorithms) on average and at the same time provide terrible predictions for single subjects. Therefore one should always check individuals with risk factor constellations for which the rival models predict

differently (see Figure 7.7). In cases where two or more rival models
have similar average performance but very different performance in
certain regions of the risk predictor space, it may be indicated to
average the predictions of the models, e.g., by means of a super
learner (Section 8.4).

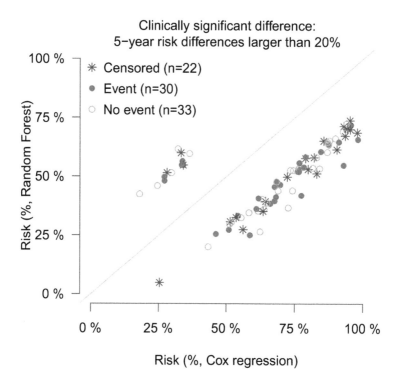

FIGURE 7.7
Oral cancer study. Scatterplot showing individual 5-year risk predictions obtained with a Cox regression model (x-axis) and a random forest model (y-
axis). Shown are only subjects outside the region of the clinically insignificant
difference in prediction, where the predicted 5-year risks of the two models
differed by more than 20%.

7. Cross-validation competition

   When a list of two or more prediction models (prediction model
   algorithms) are compared with respect to performance, cross-
   validation can select a winner based on a performance metric. This
   is readily implemented in the tuning steps of many machine learn-

ing algorithms. For example, cross-validation is used to select the hyperparameters of a random forest or the penalty of an elastic net (Section 8.2.1). In addition, a list of rival traditional regression models can be combined by cross-validation via the super learner, see Section 8.4.

8. Fallacy of prediction modeling

A cross-validation competition between two or more rival modeling algorithms immediately defines a new modeling algorithm which combines the rival modeling algorithms into a super learner (see Section 8.4). Then again, since two different super learners can be combined into a new meta algorithm, we quickly run into a circular argument.

7.5 Missing values

Missing values in the dataset should almost always be a concern [165]. When the target of the analysis is an association parameter such as an odds ratio or a hazard ratio, then it is well known that methods such as *multiple imputation* and *inverse probability weighting* can be used to reduce bias and to increase power compared to a *complete case analysis*. However, it is not so simple that multiple imputation is always better than complete case analysis, and to address the topic of this book we also need a focus on the prediction of a personalized probability. The output of a risk prediction model is more complex than an association parameter and the effect of missing values is less obvious and less studied. Another major difference to the estimation of association parameters is the setup for evaluating a risk prediction model. When the aim is to build and validate a risk prediction model, we need to deal with missing values in two places: the learning dataset and the validation dataset. In particular, we shall also address the situation where a new patient who is asking for a predicted risk has missing values in the predictor variables that are used to execute the model.

In this section, we think of missing values in the predictor variables and not so much of missing values in the outcome. Generally, not much can be learned from a subject for whom the outcome value is missing, with the important exception discussed in Chapter 5 when the outcome is not completely missing but only right-censored. The following terms describe the type of missingness:

Missing completely at random	The probability of a missing value is not related to either outcome or predictor variables.
Missing at random	The probability of a missing value is predictable by the other predictor variables and outcome.
Missing not at random	The probability of a missing value depends on the missing value and/or on other unobserved variables.

An inconvenient truth to realize is that the type of missingness can generally not be inferred from the data. Therefore, an important first step is to explore the reasons for the missing values in the dataset. This can, for example, be approached by interviewing people involved in the measurements and data collection processes. If the reason is that someone has forgotten to type a value into the computer, this will likely be *missing completely at random*. If men are more likely to tell you their body weight than women, body weight could potentially be *missing at random* if sex is a predictor. Whether it actually is *missing at random*, would depend on whether all factors (including gender) that affect the missingness of the weight value are observed. Sometimes illness severity of a patient can prohibit the collection of data such as the results of an exercise test. Here the missingness of the test result is clearly related to its unobserved latent value. This is an example of *missing not at random*.

A *complete case analysis* will simply remove all data from a subject when at least one predictor variable has a missing value. This means that having few predictor variables with a high percentage of missingness can be equally bad as having many predictor variables with few missing values in different patients. The most common form is so-called *non-monotone* missingness where the missing values are spread across variables and patients in a non-systematic way. However, when a missing value in one variable implies that the values of other variables are also missing (this part of) the missingness mechanism can be called *monotone* [174]. This is relevant, for example, when there is a time structure in the variables such that as soon as a patient has dropped out of the study, all the subsequent measurements are missing. Missing values can also occur in blocks. For example, when a blood test (or genetic test) is not performed, then all biomarker values (all genes) have missing values for this patient. Here, a cost-benefit analysis may be of interest to assess how much predictive power is lost when a time- or cost-expensive test is not performed. The consequence may be that one should build two models: one which requires the test and one which does not. The latter can be achieved in two ways; the first option is to leave out all the predictor variables corresponding to the test and the second option is to enrich the model such that the test is optional for the user (see Section 7.5.2).

Under *missing at random* and under *missing completely at random*, multiple imputation [36] and inverse probability weighting [180, 167] are principle approaches that can be helpful in the sense that they can potentially reduce the bias and increase the power compared to a complete case analysis [143]. But, under *missing not at random*, it may happen that these methods incur a bias which the complete case analysis does not have. This is because a complete case analysis can be unbiased under *missing at random* and *missing not at random* when the missingness does not depend on the outcome conditional on the predictor variables, see e.g., [180, 160].

Thinking about how missingness can possibly depend on an outcome variable is generally cumbersome, and it does not get any easier when the outcome is a right-censored time-to-event variable. If the missingness of a predictor variable "happens" at baseline, then there cannot be a direct causal effect of the outcome variable on the missingness. Hence, if the missingness depends on a time-to-event variable conditional on the observed predictor variables, this must mean that there exists an unobserved variable, such as disease burdon, which mediates the relationship. However, when the values of a predictor are collected in a retrospective manner, missingness can depend on the (right-censored) outcome in a direct causal manner. For example, it may be that a variable is only available (not missing) for those patients who survived and were not censored at the prediction horizon.

7.5.1 Missing values in the learning data

Since no real-world dataset is complete, our task is to build a risk prediction model based on a dataset with missing values in the predictor variables. In the following discussion we suppose that we have a given risk prediction model, and we refer to this model as *the substantive model*.

To begin with, the selection of predictor variables for *the substantive model* should typically consider the frequency of missingness in the data. Predictor variables with near 100% missing values should usually not be considered. Also, in order to make a useful model, one should consider how likely it is that a future patient who wants a risk prediction from the model will not be able to know the value of an important predictor variable, and how this would affect the real-life application of the model. For example, the prediction may depend on a time- or money-wise expensive test.

Next, in order to deal with the missing values, we have to specify further models, in addition to our substantive model, that relate the other variables in the dataset to each other. These additional models are called *nuisance models*. A nuisance model can be a structural model; for example, such a model could state that missingness of a variable does not depend on the other variables.

A complete case analysis implicitly requires that the missingness of the predictor variables is independent of the outcome conditional on the observed data.

A nuisance model can also be a fully parameterized regression model for the distribution of a predictor variable which allows us to predict the missing values based on the observed data.

The major approaches to deal with missing data are inverse probability weighting and multiple imputation [143]. Inverse probability weighting requires nuisance models that allow us to predict if the values are missing based on the observed data. However, in the common case where multiple predictor variables have a non-monotone missingness pattern, the development of the mathematical background for inverse probability weighting is rather recent [167, 168] and there is a lack of software. The mathematical background for multiple imputation is also not fully established, and justified mostly by computer simulation (exceptions are references [174, 62]), however, there is plenty of software to perform multiple imputation. Multiple imputation requires *nuisance models* that allow us to predict the missing values of the predictor variables based on the observed data.

Misspecification of any one of the nuisance models or the substantive model can lead to decreased prediction performance.

Imputation means to replace a missing value with a likely value. For example, to impute a value for BMI we could specify a linear regression model which relates BMI to the other predictor variables, other auxiliary variables, and the outcome. It is well known that multiple imputation analysis should condition on the outcome in order to be unbiased [133], and this is also illustrated by Figure 7.8.

In a hypothetical situation where BMI is the only predictor and the data-generating model is a Cox regression which shows an effect of BMI on survival, the simplest nuisance model for imputing missing BMI values is a normal distribution for BMI centered at the mean of the observed BMI values. However, since the survival distribution depends on BMI we can improve the nuisance model by conditioning on the survival outcome: Figure 7.8 suggests that a subject with a relatively long survival time would more likely have a larger BMI than a subject with a relatively short survival time. However, in particular because the survival outcome is also right-censored, it is not so easy to specify a regression model which parameterizes how BMI (or any other predictor variable) depends on the pair of the censored survival time and the censoring indicator. The solution of Bartlett et al., called the SMCFCS algorithm [16], is appealing and Bayesian. It is Bayesian not only because the developers use the Bayes formula inside their algorithm to trade the dependence of the predictor variable on the outcome into a dependence of the outcome on the predictor variable. In this way, they accomplish a multiple imputation algorithm that is consistent with the substantive model. The SMCFCS algorithm [15] works for various outcomes and substantive models. For our purposes, it is worth noting that it works for logistic regression models, i.e., uncensored binary outcome, and Cox regression models, i.e., right-censored survival outcome. In the presence of competing risks, the substantive model SMCFCS specifies two cause-specific Cox regression models: one for the hazard rate of the cause of interest and one for the hazard rate of the competing risk. In addition to the substantive model, SMCFCS relies on a parametric regres-

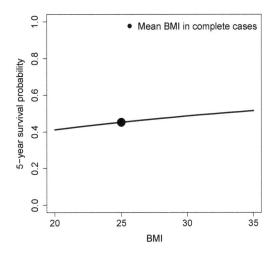

FIGURE 7.8

Suppose the substantive model is a Cox regression model which shows that
the 5-year survival probability increases with increasing BMI as shown in
the figure. Without conditioning on the outcome, we simply impute missing
BMI values for every one from a normal distribution with mean given by the
mean BMI in the complete cases. When the 5-year survival probability is an
increasing function of BMI as in the figure this imputed value (the black dot
on the line) is systematically too large for subjects with BMI below 25 and
systematically lowlarge for subjects with BMI above 25.

sion model for each predictor variable that has missing values. As with any other multiple imputation algorithm, SMCFCS repeats imputation multiple times and returns multiple datasets in which the missing values are replaced by values drawn under a random distribution which is dictated by the set of nuisance models. In the remainder of this section, we provide some insights based on computer simulation on the effect of missing values in the learning data on the prediction performance when the prediction model is based on SMCFCS. For the purpose of illustration we simulate a large validation set (n=10,000) which does not have missing values and use it to estimate the prediction performance parameters (AUC, IPA).

We simulate biomarker values from a normal distribution in such a way that low and high values are associated with a high risk of a binary outcome (uncensored) as shown in panel A of Figure 7.9. In addition to the biomarker, we also simulate a binary variable (we think of gender) and a uniform variable with values between 30 and 90 (we think of age). Both these predictor variables have an effect on the risk of the outcome event and also an effect on the distribution of the biomarker, and neither has missing values. The data-generating model consists of a linear regression model for the distribution of the biomarker and a logistic regression model with 4 variables (the biomarker, the squared biomarker, gender, age) each having an additive effect on the linear predictor. Furthermore, a logistic regression model is used to simulate missing biomarker values under varying constellations to achieve *missing at random, missing completely at random* and *missing not at random*, respectively. The other panels of Figure 7.9 (B-D) show our simulated missingness mechanisms under the three scenarios.

We show results from 200 simulated datasets for each fixed parameter constellation. The number of imputed datasets has a clear effect on the prediction performance (Figure 7.10). The more imputations, the better the prediction performance. In this specific simulation scenario, it looks as if 10 imputations are sufficient in the sense that more imputations do not further improve the prediction performance.

However, for the purpose of having a model which should be applied to individual patients in real life, it is not sufficient to consider prediction performance on average in order to judge if 10 or 20 imputations are sufficient. What is to be avoided is that any single patient receives a predicted probability from the model that suffers from a considerable random seed effect. Figure 7.11 shows that the individual predicted risks still vary too much even with 20 imputations. The effect would be that some patients, by chance, would receive a predicted risk that is off by as much as 20%. The figure also shows, that in the particular dataset, 200 imputations were sufficient to have consistently predicted risks under two different random seeds. To be thorough, we should define a convergence criterion to define the number of multiple imputations at which the algorithm has converged.

In Figure 7.12 we show the average prediction performance of the complete case analysis and the multiple imputation analysis in our specific *missing at*

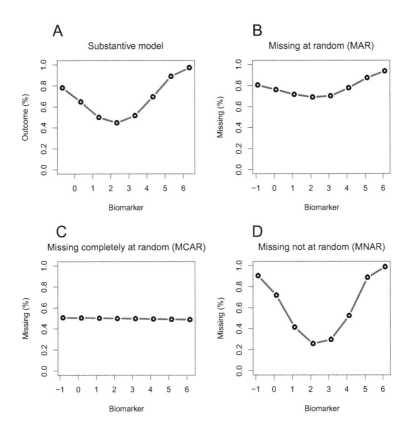

FIGURE 7.9
Illustration of the simulation setting where a biomarker affects the outcome risk in a non-linear fashion (panel A). Panel B shows the scenario where the probability of a missing biomarker value depends on the observed variables (outcome, age, gender). Panel C shows the scenario where the probability of a missing biomarker value is independent of all other variables. Panel D shows the scenario where the probability of a missing biomarker value depends on the biomarker value itself.

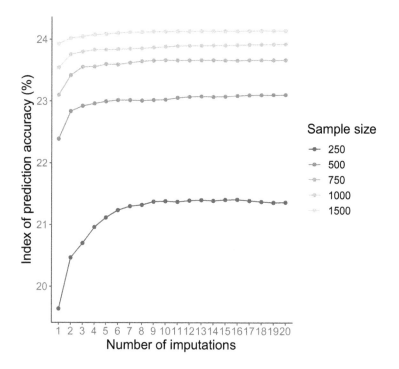

FIGURE 7.10
Results of empirical studies (200 simulated learning datasets) under a varying
number of imputations (x-axis) in our *missing at random* setting. The index
of prediction accuracy is increasing with an increasing number of imputations
across all sample sizes. The prediction performance parameters are computed
in a huge validation dataset (n=20,000) without missing values.

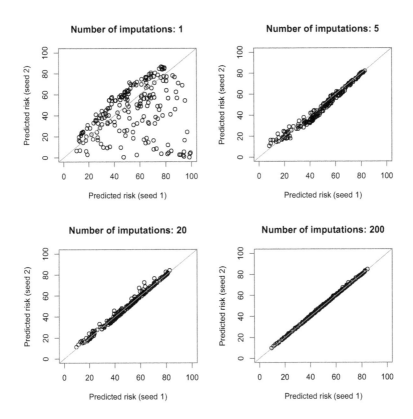

FIGURE 7.11
A risk prediction model based on logistic regression fitted with multiple imputation on a single training dataset (n=200, $\sim$ 50% missing values) using
two different random seeds. Shown are predicted risks in a single independent
validation set.

random setting (Figure 7.9, Panel B). We see that the complete case analysis has a huge problem when the missingness depends on the outcome, also with low or moderate missingness.

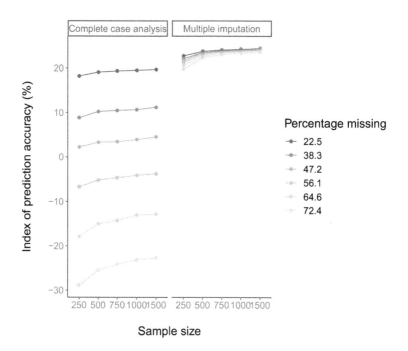

FIGURE 7.12
Results of empirical studies in our specific *missing at random* setting where the index of prediction accuracy is calculated based on an independent validation dataset without missing values (n=20,000). Shown are averages across 200 simulated learning datasets where in each we applied both complete case analysis and multiple imputation analysis. The sample size of the learning datasets varies across the values 250, 500, 750, 1000, 1500.

In the *missing completely at random* setting (Figure 7.13), the multiple imputation analysis scores higher IPA values than the complete case analysis. In our specific *missing not at random* setting, the performance of the complete case analysis is comparable to that of the multiple imputation analysis, except perhaps in the small sample sizes where the multiple imputation analysis scores higher IPA values. However, recall that in general under *missing not at random*, the multiple imputation analysis can be biased (leading to a lower IPA) when the complete case analysis is not.

Also, it is important to note that in all the empirical studies presented so far, the substantive model and the nuisance models used by multiple imputation analysis were correctly specified. In Figure 7.14 we compare the predictive performance of two multiple imputation analyses, one based on correctly specified models and one based on misspecified models (omitted quadratic effect of the biomarker). In this specific case, there is a tradeoff. In small sample sizes, the misspecified multiple imputation analysis scores higher IPA values than the correctly specified imputation analysis, and in large sample sizes, the correctly specified imputation analysis has higher prediction performance than the misspecified multiple imputation analysis.

7.5.2 Missing values in the validation data

The aim of a validation analysis for a prediction model is to inform future patients (users of the model) about the expected performance of the model. We distinguish the following two tasks. The first task is to have the validation analysis deal with missing values in the validation dataset. The second task is to enrich the model such that the input values of some of the predictor variables become optional for the user of the model. That is, if the user of the model cannot provide the value of one or several predictors, ideally, then the model should still be able to provide a predicted risk. It seems clear that a solution to the second task brings with it a solution for the first task: by using the validation dataset which contains missing values we simulate how the model performs in the realistic setting where some patients do not provide all the predictor values. Obviously, this makes most sense when the missingness in the validation dataset resembles the expected missingness in the future users of the model.

Figure 7.15 shows an example where the predictor variable %free PSA is optional. In addition to the risk of high-grade prostate cancer within 4 years, predicted as 8% when %free PSA is unknown, the patient is also informed that the predicted risk would be 50% in case of an extremely low %free PSA value and only 5% in case of an extremely high %free PSA value. This particular example indicates that if an important predictor variable has a missing value, like %free PSA in the context of prostate cancer, then the risk prediction would potentially change a lot had the value been available. In such a situation, it may be most useful to provide the user with the range of predicted risks and a recommendation to obtain the measurement to increase the accuracy. However, if one has a highly accurate model to predict %free PSA based on the available data, then the risk prediction model can be enriched and provide reliable risk predictions even if the %free PSA is missing. This is more complicated in the common case were multiple predictor variables may have missing values.

It remains to discuss alternative ways to enrich a risk prediction model

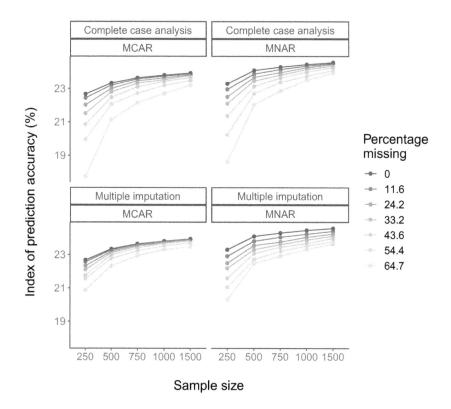

FIGURE 7.13
Results of empirical studies of our specific *missing completely at random* and *missing not at random* settings where the index of prediction accuracy is calculated based on an independent validation dataset without missing values (n=20,000). Shown are averages across 200 simulated learning datasets where, in each, we applied both complete case analysis and multiple imputation analysis. The sample size of the learning datasets varies across the values 250, 500, 750, 1000, 1500.

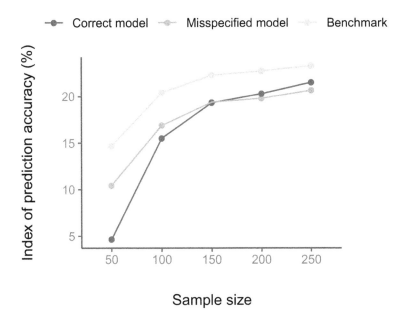

FIGURE 7.14
Results of empirical studies of our *missing at random* setting where the index of prediction accuracy is calculated based on an independent validation dataset without missing values (n=20,000). Shown are averages across 200 simulated learning datasets from the setting where about 56% of the values of the biomarker were missing. In each simulated dataset, we applied a multiple imputation analysis using correctly specified substantive and nuisance models and a second multiple imputation analysis which wrongly omits the quadratic effect of the biomarker. To obtain the benchmark, we applied a logistic regression model in a copy of the dataset without missing values.

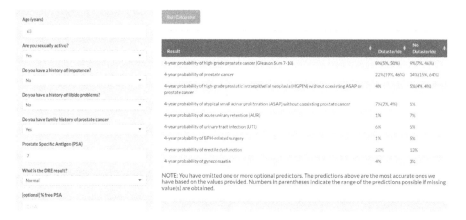

FIGURE 7.15
Example Internet calculator where user obtains a result even though no value
is provided for an important predictor (%free PSA). The user also sees the
potential range of predicted probabilities if the missing variable value is obtained.

such that the model can be applied even when some predictor variables have
missing values. A general idea is to replace the missing values with expected
values and then to apply the risk prediction model. However, if simply the
average value of the learning data is used as "expected value," the prediction performance suffers [105]. A more sophisticated approach is the one-step
SWEEP method [128] which works in generalized linear regression models.
The basic idea is to consider submodels for all possible missing value patterns
such that the regression parameters corresponding to the predictor variables
with missing values are all set to zero. Thus, the model is enriched by submodels such that the predicted risk for a new patient is obtained with the
submodel that contains only the predictor variables for which the new patient
can provide values. It is argued that fitting all the submodels in the learning dataset is computationally expensive and instead, the SWEEP operator
is used to obtain an approximation of the submodels [128]. Nowadays, the
computational burden may be less problematic in most settings. However, a
real challenge that was not discussed in [128] is that one needs to specify all
these submodels. It can be time-consuming to optimize variable selection and
functional form selection for them all, and also there is a risk of miscalibration
when important predictor variables are not included. An alternative way to
enrich the risk prediction model is to build imputation models for the pattern
of missing values that allow one to predict likely values of the optional variables, i.e., the variables that have missing values, given the observed data of
the future patient (user of the model). This approach has the advantage that
the same model with all predictors is run for all new patients, and no submod-

els are needed. However, various additional models are needed to handle the imputation. But, for the purpose of predicting the risk of a future patient, the additional models may not depend on the outcome. In a specific simulation scenario, Jannsen et al. [105] showed that multiple imputation in conjunction with the full model can outperform the prediction performance achieved by submodels. In order to use multiple imputation, Jannsen et al. [105] require that the learning data (they call it the derivation set) are processed together with the new patient's data. This is a cumbersome procedure since the training data must be uploaded to the risk calculator. However, technically it is not necessary to save the learning data to make some variables optional; it is sufficient to provide models that allow the computer to calculate the most likely value for each optional predictor variable based on the provided predictor variables.

7.6   Time-varying coefficient models

Standard Cox regression models rely on a proportional hazard assumption, which means that the regression coefficients (i.e., the weights given to the predictor variables) are constant in time. Of course, there are many ways to relax this assumption [129] and in particular, for categorical predictor variables, all that is needed is to stratify the baseline hazard function. Using the methods of this chapter it is straightforward to perform a head-to-head comparison of a Cox regression model that assumes proportional hazards to another model which does not have this assumption with respect to prediction performance. Furthermore, there is the possibility to compare with a stopped Cox regression model [179].

In Section 4.1.2 we showed how to stop the event time at the prediction time horizon. We argued that this is sometimes useful, for example, in the context of a Cox proportional hazard model. The intuition is that events that occur after the prediction time horizon do not help to improve the predicted risks. However, stopping Cox regression may or may not improve predictive performance. The following illustration shows an example where it does not improve the prediction performance. We consider the complete cases of the oral cancer study and compare an unstopped Cox regression model with a Cox regression model which is stopped after 5 years using the *leave-one-out bootstrap* (Section 7.4.3) based on 200 splits (could be 2000 splits).

```
# R-code
oc.cc$survtime.5years <- pmin(oc.cc$survtime,60) # stop time after
    5 years
oc.cc$survstatus.5years <- oc.cc$survstatus # take a copy
oc.cc[oc.cc$survtime>60,]$survstatus.5years <- 0 # reset status
fit1 <- cph(Surv(survtime,survstatus)~rcs(age,3)+tumorthickness+
```

```
                gender+tobacco+deep.invasion+race+x.posnodes+tumormaxdimension+
                vascular.invasion,
                     data=oc.cc, x=TRUE, y=TRUE, surv=TRUE)
       fit2 <- cph(Surv(survtime.5years,survstatus.5years)~rcs(age,3)+
                tumorthickness+gender+tobacco+deep.invasion+race+x.posnodes+
                tumormaxdimension+vascular.invasion,
                     data=oc.cc, x=TRUE, y=TRUE, surv=TRUE)
       x <- Score(list("Unstopped"=fit1,"Stopped.5yrs"=fit2),
                data=oc.cc,
                formula=Surv(survtime,survstatus)~1,
                times=60,
                summary=c("IPA"),
                null.model=1,
                split.method="loob",
                B=200) # could be 2000
```

times	Model	AUC (%)	Brier (%)	IPA
60	Null model	50.0 [50.0;50.0]	24.9 [19.7;30.1]	0.0
60	Unstopped	75.2 [71.1;79.3]	20.1 [15.6;24.6]	19.2
60	Stopped.5yrs	74.9 [70.8;78.9]	20.2 [15.7;24.7]	18.8

In this particular example, artificial censoring leads to loss of prediction performance: the stopped model has a lower AUC, higher Brier score, and a lower IPA than the unstopped model.

7.7   Time-varying predictor variables

We first need to distinguish between variables that are under the control of either the doctor or the patient, e.g., treatment/intervention, versus those that are simply measured, e.g., a blood test. The reason we make this distinction is that it is possible to provide predictions conditional upon whether the patient is starting and continuing with an intervention such as treatment, but it certainly does not make sense to provide the prediction that depends on the future value of a blood test. In summary, we can base our predictions on any values measured today or prior to today, but we can only condition on future variables that are under our control.

While it is straightforward to fit, for example, a Cox regression model that depends on time-varying covariates, it is not obvious how to apply the model on new patients in order to inform about risks. The problem is that the predicted risk should be communicated to a new patient at time zero, and at that time, the values that a time-varying variable may take later on are not yet available. The attraction of a landmark analysis [178] (Section 6.4.2) is that it keeps pushing time zero out to today. Landmarking is valuable because it has the ability to use the history of any longitudinal marker, such as a series of blood tests, in addition to the current value of the marker, to improve the prediction. There may be information in whether a certain marker has increased or decreased since the last measurement. The key here is that the information is available by looking back in time from the landmark time point (Figure 7.16). See Section 3.4.4 for an example. There the repeated measurements of PSA within the last two years used to calculate the PSA doubling time, which is predictive of outcome in prostate cancer patients.

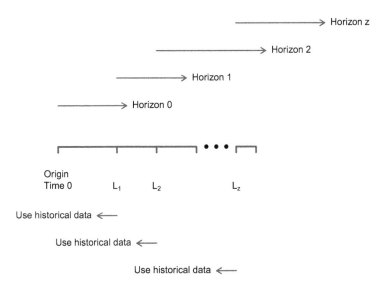

FIGURE 7.16
Scheme for landmark analysis. Historical data refer to covariate history.

In clinical use, the predictions can be updated whenever any predictor variable changes value. Revised predictions are provided as patients return for follow-up appointments, and updated values for their predictor variables, e.g., blood test, are used to update the risk prediction since the last visit (landmark time point). A difficulty for the modeler is that the time span between blood tests is not typically the same for different patients who are often following irregular measurement schemes that may even depend on the development of the disease. For example, a patient would ask for a visit in case of new symptoms. Consequently, many of the available modeling options implicitly assume that the time-varying predictor variables, e.g., the blood markers, are changing in a predictable manner between visits.

There are several sophisticated modeling approaches that can accommodate time-varying variables. One such approach is multi-state modeling [7, 177]. Broadly, this approach utilizes discrete states through which a patient may transition (Figure 7.17).

"Transition" means going from one state to another, and a Cox regression model can then be used to estimate the transition hazard rate conditional on the current predictor variable history. These transition rates can be combined to derive a personalized predictive probability at each landmark time point for a given prediction time horizon. However, the formulas to implement this approach are complicated and difficult to implement, but see reference [51]. Therefore, a more simplistic approach [177] is to fit a separate prediction model at each landmark time point using the subjects at-risk at that time (at-risk = alive and event-free and not censored). If there are insufficient data for these many landmark models, it may be possible to make use of the connection between a sequence of binary regression models and complex survival analysis [106, 56]. Another fruitful class of models that can provide time dynamic prediction models are so-called joint models for the joint distribution of longitudinal predictor variables and survival outcome [150, 169].

Each landmark model can be assessed for prediction accuracy described in Chapters 5 and 6. This can produce a time series of predictive accuracy [27] which can be visualized by a plot of accuracy versus landmark time for a fixed prediction time horizon, see e.g., reference [46] for an example.

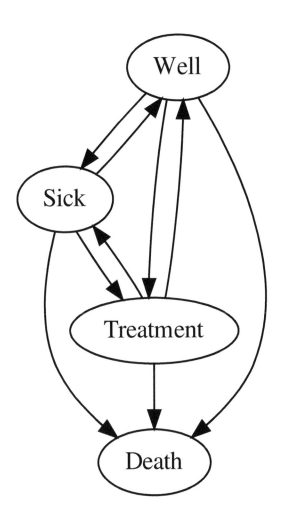

FIGURE 7.17
Generic multi-state model. At any time, the patient is in one of these states.
Arrows indicate possible transitions that may depend on patient characteristics and history of longitudinal markers and hence need to be modeled.

8

Can't the computer just take care of all of this?

You might think that there is one correct way to build a statistical prediction model. This is not true, but different strategies have their strengths and weaknesses. Moreover, some strategies should not be used because they are dominated by other strategies. For example, it is common to see the researcher split several biomarkers (continuous variables) into binary variables using the cutpoints he likes, e.g., at the median values. Then he counts the number of risk factors that a patient has and groups patients by this number of risk factors. For example, the highest risk group may have more than four risk factors. The results will be outperformed by any of the strategies described in this chapter. Another example of an inferior method is the stepwise variable selection with backward elimination being its most commonly seen form. It is inferior in the sense that advanced algorithms that incorporate cross-validation to control overfitting, such as the LASSO (Section 8.2.1), usually outperform backward elimination in a head-to-head comparison.

What is the difference between traditional regression models and machine learning? A useful reference for this is Breiman's view on the two cultures [32]. In a logistic regression model or Cox regression model, inference on association parameters such as odds ratios and hazard ratios is valid under the assumption of a completely pre-specified regression model. However, it is not always feasible to completely pre-specify which variables should enter the model and in what way, and the more the data are used to select the model in general and the predictor variables in particular, the less correct becomes the naive inference, which ignores the selection. As a result of using the same data for model selection and inference, we see inflated type-I errors, i.e., systematically too small p-values and too narrow confidence intervals [87]. But not only the inference about association parameters suffers from the form of overfitting, also the predictions for yet unseen patients may become systematically too high or too low. In this chapter, we advocate the use of cross-validation as a mandatory tool also for prediction model building. Nested layers of cross-validation are needed when we use internal cross-validation (Section 7.4) to assess the prediction performance of a modeling algorithm which uses cross-validation to build the model.

At this point, you should have an idea of how cross-validation works (Section 7.4) and which prediction performance metrics are available to guide prediction modeling (Chapters 5, 6). You may have skipped ahead to look for the quick fix to your problem. However, just trying to find an automated solution without understanding what is happening can cause problems that you do not even realize, and of course, if you put garbage in, you will get garbage out, no matter how fancy your method is.

We now discuss the recommended approaches to building statistical prediction models. They are tentatively listed in order of demand for sample size relative to the number of predictors.

There is a tradeoff between the sample size and the number of data-dependent decisions.

With a small sample size either the model complexity is reduced, or expert knowledge and external data should replace some of the data-dependent decisions, or both. We go from the setting where the computer does not make a single decision (Section 8.1) to the extreme where the computer makes almost all decisions (Sections 8.3, 8.4). In between we have Section 8.2 where a single layer of cross-validation is applied to assist things like variable selection, number of knots for cubic splines and selection of penalty parameters. In order to use any of the approaches in a meaningful way, the data have to be prepared (see Chapter 3) in an unsupervised fashion, i.e., without looking at the association between predictor variables and outcome.

8.1 Zero layers of cross-validation

Suppose the ambition is to build the prediction model without using cross-validation at all. Doing so requires a regression model where the researcher makes all modeling decisions by using external knowledge provided by a subject matter expert and the literature. There is a tradeoff here. If you do indeed make all the decisions before looking at the data, you may run into problems (Section 8.1.1). Note that looking at the data, blinded to the outcome variable, is okay (see Section 8.1.2). For example, you might decide to merge categories with sparse data. The key is to remain unsupervised, blinded to the outcome.

8.1.1 What may happen if you do not look at the data

A common problem is related to collinearity (Section 2.5.7). The following model attempts to include all available variables of the IVF learning dataset in a logistic regression model.

```
# R-code
fit <- glm(ohss~ cyclelen + bmi + weight + age + ant.foll + fsh +
    smoking + no.cig.d + ovolume,data=ivftrain,family="binomial")
```

```
Error in 'contrasts<-'('*tmp*', value = contr.funs[1 + isOF[nn]]) :
  contrasts can be applied only to factors with 2 or more levels
```

This is one variant of a very common error. The general explanation is that given the other variables, there is at least one variable without residual variability in the data. In the present case, it simply means that given the number of cigarettes per day (*no.cig.d*) there is no variability in the binary smoking status (*smoking*), in particular for all patients with *no.cig.d=0*, the smoking status has the value "*no.*" The next thing to do is figure out which variable is causing this problem. Then maybe removing the variable brings you to the next problem. The following model has removed the offending variable (*smoking*).

```
# R-code
fit <- glm(ohss~ cyclelen + bmi + weight + age + ant.foll + fsh +
    no.cig.d + ovolume,data=ivftrain,family="binomial")
fit
```

```
Warning messages:
1: glm.fit: algorithm did not converge
2: glm.fit: fitted probabilities numerically 0 or 1 occurred

Call:  glm(formula = ohss ~ cyclelen + bmi + weight + age + ant.foll +
    fsh + no.cig.d + ovolume, family = "binomial", data = ivftrain)

Coefficients:
(Intercept)      cyclelen            bmi         weight          age
  -2351.152        42.832        240.565        -65.031       -0.282
    ant.foll           fsh       no.cig.d        ovolume
      28.435      -133.363        -20.664         15.137

Degrees of Freedom: 50 Total (i.e. Null);  42 Residual
  (123 observations deleted due to missingness)
Null Deviance:             57.9
Residual Deviance: 0.00000008106          AIC: 18
```

We see here that the computer has deleted the majority of the data. In general, this means that there are missing values in at least one variable. In this specific case, it means that we lack one important data preparation step, namely, we did not code non-smokers as zero in the number of cigarettes per day variable. In fact, zero was coded as missing. The technical problems (warnings) are removed when we build our full model by substituting the binary smoking status variable for the number of cigarettes per day variable.

```
# R-code
fit <- glm(ohss~ cyclelen + bmi + weight + age + ant.foll + fsh +
    smoking + ovolume,data=ivftrain,family="binomial")
fit
```

```
Call:  glm(formula = ohss ~ cyclelen + bmi + weight + age + ant.foll +
    fsh + smoking + ovolume, family = "binomial", data = ivftrain)

Coefficients:
(Intercept)     cyclelen           bmi        weight           age
  -6.332167     0.114296      0.083451     -0.013667     -0.046635
    ant.foll          fsh     smokingYes       ovolume
    0.133106     0.001237     -0.954389      0.023959

Degrees of Freedom: 173 Total (i.e. Null);   165 Residual
Null Deviance:              220.1
Residual Deviance: 167.7           AIC: 185.7
```

8.1.2   Unsupervised modeling steps

Suppose you have an insufficient amount of data to fit a regression model even after proper data preparation. This can happen with any number of predictor variables, but it will always happen when you have a so-called high-dimensional problem where the number of predictors exceeds the number of patients in the purpose dataset. There are a few techniques that ignore the outcome variable and may still help you to move forward with variable selection. Since they do not consider the outcome variable, they are called unsupervised and may not need cross-validation. One such dimension reduction technique is called principal components analysis (PCA). PCA is useful for reducing the number of continuous predictor variables in the model while retaining much of the information content of the original continuous predictors.

> *The total variance is the sum of the purpose data variances of all predictor variables.*

Principal components are linear combinations of the original continuous predictors constructed such that they explain as much as possible of the total variance of the data (excluding the outcome and the categorical predictors). The total variance is the sum of the variances of the continuous predictors. The principal components are new variables that are uncorrelated with each other. The modeler needs to decide the number of principal components to put in the final model. The more principal components you include, the higher fraction of the total variance is explained by these principal components. To select the number of principal components, one option is to fix a threshold of the percent total variance explained by the principal components, e.g., 95%, and use as many new variables (principal components) as needed to achieve that threshold. Then, one can replace the original predictors with the new variables (principal components). Alternatively, one can visualize the results of PCA, e.g., by a graph of the kind shown in Figure 8.1. Such a graph can guide variable selection whereby we could choose one of the variables when its arrow is superimposed over another variable's arrow. Note that since we are unsupervised at this stage, we cannot tell which selection leads to the better prediction model, but in this way we can potentially avoid collinearity.

In our in vitro fertilization study we apply PCA to the 7 continuous predictors (cycle length, BMI, body weight, age, number of antral follicles, hormone FSH, and ovarian volume).

```
# R-code
library(FactoMineR)
Vars <- ivftrain[,c("cyclelen","bmi","weight","age","ant.foll","fsh
   ","ovolume")]
fit <- PCA(Vars,scale.unit=TRUE,ncp=5,graph=FALSE)
plot(fit,new.plot=FALSE,choix="var")
```

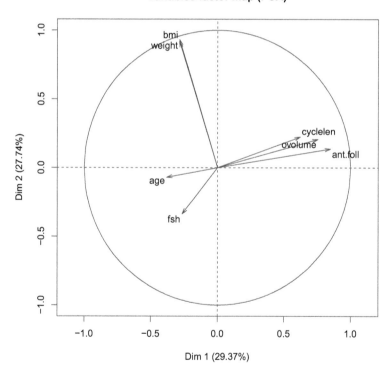

FIGURE 8.1
In vitro fertilization study. Principal components analysis of the continuous predictor variables.

Figure 8.1 shows the first two principal components. They explain 29.13%

and 26.64% of the purpose dataset, respectively. Figure 8.1 suggests that you probably only need BMI or body weight but not both. There is a similar suggestion regarding the ovarian volume and cycle length and the number of antral follicles. These are merely suggestions as we are not looking at further dimensions in the data. The variables age, and hormone FSH seem to pull the first two principal components in different directions.

Another example of an unsupervised modeling step is to use restricted cubic splines for a continuous predictor variable (Section 4.3.2). This is a very useful technique for allowing a continuous variable to have a non-linear effect. For example, many routine blood tests have a normal range such that either low or high values may indicate high risk. The challenges here are which continuous variables to add the splines to and how many knots to use for each. More knots are needed to describe more flexible relationships. Since we are unsupervised, we must rely upon quantiles of the distribution for knot placement or use an expert's opinion regarding the biology in order to choose the number and/or placement of knots. However, if the expert indicates a very complicated relationship and hence suggests many knots, the sample size may still limit the feasibility. In practice, simply using 3 knots placed at the quartiles works pretty well.

In our in vitro fertilization study, we could, for example, use restricted cubic splines with 3 knots for all the continuous predictor variables. In the context of our logistic regression model, this means that we spend two regression coefficients (odds ratios) instead of one for each of the continuous predictor variables.

```
# R-code
fit <- lrm(ohss~ smoking+ rcs(cyclelen,3) + rcs(bmi,3) + rcs(weight
    ,3) + rcs(age,3) + rcs(ant.foll,3) + rcs(fsh,3) + rcs(ovolume
    ,3),data=ivftrain)
coef(fit)
```

Intercept	smoking=Yes	cyclelen	cyclelen'	bmi
-17.90578645	-0.99374250	0.29603566	-0.26420685	0.45630635
bmi'	weight	weight'	age	age'
-0.57238334	-0.14498317	0.17945134	0.08137955	-0.19704648
ant.foll	ant.foll'	fsh	fsh'	ovolume
0.29285379	-0.23105238	-0.19666265	0.34663232	0.16113176
ovolume'				
-0.12350439				

However, when the sample size is relatively small (as in our in vitro fertilization study) and the number of continuous predictor variables that are included with a restricted cubic spline is relatively large (as in our vitro fertilization study) data overfitting may occur and may lead to unreliable risk predictions. A possible way to treat this problem is shrinkage [120], where the magnitude of all estimated regression coefficients is shrunk toward zero by means of a penalty term:

```
# R-code
fit <- lrm(ohss~ smoking+ rcs(cyclelen,3) + rcs(bmi,3) + rcs(weight
    ,3) + rcs(age,3) + rcs(ant.foll,3) + rcs(fsh,3) + rcs(ovolume
    ,3),
        data=ivftrain,
        penalty=10)
coef(fit)
```

```
    Intercept    smoking=Yes        cyclelen       cyclelen'              bmi
-4.9449316880 -0.4495863903   0.0872247773   0.0445293815    0.0185225105
         bmi'         weight         weight'             age             age'
-0.0121167458 -0.0009663036   0.0069589538  -0.0040883373   -0.0764208096
     ant.foll      ant.foll'             fsh            fsh'          ovolume
 0.0641424203   0.0325110088  -0.0626046024   0.0568336246    0.0575561473
     ovolume'
-0.0119890296
```

The effect on the risk predictions of individual patients is that they are shrunk toward the total prevalence of the event (Figure 8.2).

In the test dataset of the in vitro fertilization study, the logistic regression model with ridge penalty 10 outperforms the unpenalized model.

```
# R-code
fit1 <- lrm(ohss~ smoking+ rcs(cyclelen,3) + rcs(bmi,3) + rcs(
    weight,3) + rcs(age,3) + rcs(ant.foll,3) + rcs(fsh,3) + rcs(
    ovolume,3),
        data=ivftrain,penalty=0)
fit2 <- lrm(ohss~ smoking+ rcs(cyclelen,3) + rcs(bmi,3) + rcs(
    weight,3) + rcs(age,3) + rcs(ant.foll,3) + rcs(fsh,3) + rcs(
    ovolume,3),
        data=ivftrain,
        penalty=1)
x <- Score(list(unpenalized=fit1,penalized=fit2),data=ivftest,
    formula=ohss~1)
summary(x,what="score")
```

```
$score
          Model          AUC (%)          Brier (%)
1:  Null model            50.0 21.2 [17.6;24.7]
2: unpenalized 82.6 [74.7;90.6] 15.7 [12.0;19.4]
3:   penalized 86.6 [79.5;93.6] 14.2 [11.0;17.4]
```

However, it is *a priori* unclear how much shrinkage one should apply – and this is not a case where a subject matter expert can help. So, in order to find the final model we should apply cross-validation of the training dataset to choose the penalty parameter which maximizes the expected prediction performance in future patients.

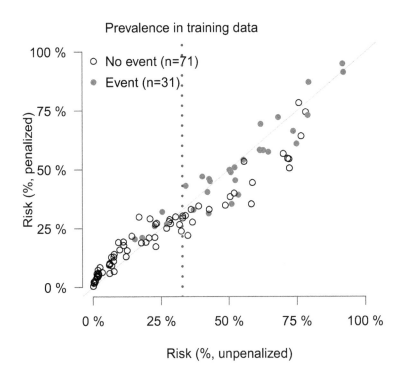

FIGURE 8.2
In vitro fertilization study. Risk predictions are shrunk toward the prevalence by the penalized fit compared to the unpenalized fit: predicted risks above (below) the training set prevalence (32.8%) are systematically more often below (above) the diagonal.

8.1.3   Final model

Once all data-related problems are removed (no errors or warnings from the
software), the unsupervised modeling strategy yields a final model. An important characteristic of this strategy is that we do not try to further improve
the final model. Considering a model goodness-of-fit test, test for interactions
between the predictor variables, or a similar attempt to tweak the model involving the outcome, would require another layer of cross-validation to control
overfitting.

In our in vitro fertilization study we could end up with the following model:

```
# R-code
fit <- glm(ohss~ cyclelen + bmi + weight + age + ant.foll + fsh +
    smoking + ovolume,data=ivftrain,family="binomial")
publish(fit)
```

Variable	Units	OddsRatio	CI.95	p-value
cyclelen		1.12	[0.93;1.36]	0.24313
bmi		1.09	[0.84;1.41]	0.52528
weight		0.99	[0.91;1.07]	0.74881
age		0.95	[0.85;1.07]	0.40985
ant.foll		1.14	[1.07;1.22]	¡ 0.0001
fsh		1.00	[0.79;1.28]	0.99204
smoking	No	Ref		
	Yes	0.39	[0.16;0.95]	0.03756
ovolume		1.02	[0.90;1.17]	0.72659

This model can be used to predict ovarian hyperstimulation syndrome
in new patients. We ignore the p-values of the odds ratios because they are
not directly related to prediction performance (Section 2.7.2). Instead, we
calculate the area under the ROC curve and the Brier score.

8.2   One layer of cross-validation

It is the natural desire of the researcher to build the best model. We describe
ways of tuning the model to hopefully increase prediction performance. Note
that these tuning methods involve the outcome – they are "supervised" – and
thus require cross-validation as part of the modeling algorithm to avoid data
overfitting. In this section, we will explore some commonly applied and well-
known modeling steps and wrap them up in a single layer of cross-validation.
It is important to note that an outer layer of cross-validation is needed to evaluate the performance of such a modeling algorithm (see Section 7.4.6). This
means that in each split of the data, the whole modeling algorithm, including its own internal cross-validation variable and hyperparameter selection, is

applied to the learning set in order to predict the outcome of the subjects in the corresponding test set.

8.2.1 Penalized regression

We consider one of the standard regression models described in Chapter 4 and Section 8.1, i.e., logistic regression for binary uncensored outcome, Cox regression for censored survival outcome, and, for a competing risk outcome, either a combination of cause-specific Cox regression models, or a Fine-Gray regression model. General reasons for fear of overfitting are too many predictor variables or too low sample size/event rate (c.f., Figure 8.3).

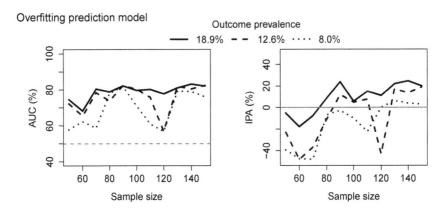

FIGURE 8.3
Simulation result obtained by fitting a logistic regression model with 10 co-variates (5 binary, 5 continuous) to small learning datasets where small is relative to the prevalence of the outcome. Shown are results calculated with a huge (n=50,000) validation set. The results are obtained with a single learning dataset for each sample size. Even though the logistic regression model is correctly specified, and the AUC is always above the magic 50%, we see that the IPA is negative for small sample sizes in particular when the outcome prevalence is low. This indicates that the null model, which ignores the 10 covariates and predicts the outcome prevalence of the learning dataset outperforms the logistic regression model. The interpretation is that the logistic regression model is overfitting the data.

Specific reasons for data overfitting are, for example, when there are many experimental predictors, i.e., predictor variables without established effects, or when the effects of continuous predictor variables are modeled in a flexible way, e.g., by restricted cubic splines. The expert knowledge approach would simplify the model, for example, by reducing the number of variables, without looking at the data. However, sometimes we believe in a more complex model but do not have sufficient data/events to fit it in a reliable way. An extreme situation occurs when we have more predictor variables than subjects in the dataset.

> *The likelihood function describes the probability to observe the data under the model. Maximum likelihood is a procedure used to estimate the regression coefficients of standard regression models.*

In this so-called high-dimensional setting, the standard maximum likelihood cannot be used to estimate the model. If we want to pursue a complex model, the general philosophy is to learn as much as possible from the data, but not too much. This can be achieved by the use of cross-validation.

Penalized maximum likelihood estimation adds a penalty term to the likelihood function. The penalty term has a shrinkage effect on the estimated regression coefficients [43, 44]. Corresponding methods are developed and implemented for generalized linear models including logistic regression [69] and Cox regression [80, 162]. Important special cases are ridge regression [99], which was developed for correlated predictor variables, the LASSO [171] which aims at variable selection, and the elastic net which combines the two [190]. While ridge regression shrinks the regression coefficients toward zero, LASSO also eliminates the ones that get very close to zero, i.e., some of the shrunk coefficients are exactly zero, and the elastic net combines the penalty term of the LASSO with the penalty term of the ridge regression.

Shrinkage often improves prediction accuracy [89]. To illustrate this, we should discuss what happens with the individualized risk predictions when penalized maximum likelihood is used, instead of unpenalized maximum likelihood, to estimate the parameters of a regression model. But, first we describe what happens to the regression parameter estimates. Consider a predictor variable that has no effect (given the other predictor variables). In this case, the corresponding population parameter, i.e., the odds ratio in a logistic regression or the hazard ratio in a Cox regression model, has the value 1. Penalization has a shrinkage effect on the estimated odds ratios (or hazard ratios) in the sense that the odds ratios (or hazard ratios) of all predictor variables have a value which is systematically closer to the value 1 (meaning no effect) compared to the unpenalized fit of a logistic regression model (or Cox regression model).

Table 8.1 illustrates the effect of shrinkage on the hazard ratios in penalized Cox regression models fitted to the training dataset of the oral cancer study. For the purpose of illustration, three different penalty parameter combinations were fixed at arbitrarily chosen values. Specifically, the value 3 for ridge regression, the value 4 for LASSO, and the values (1.5, 2.5) for the elastic net.

```
# R-code
```

```
library(penalized)
form <- Surv(survtime,survstatus)~ age + tumorthickness +
    genderMale + tobaccoNever + deep.invasionYes + siteFloor.of.
    Mouth + siteHard.Palate + siteLower.Gum + siteRetromolar.
    Trigone + siteTongue + siteUpper.Gum + raceNonCauc + x.posnodes
    + tumormaxdimension + vascular.invasionYes
# Elastic net
fit.elnet <- penalized(form, data=octrain.dummy, model="cox",
            lambda1=1.5, lambda2=2.5) # L1 and L2 penalty
# LASSO
fit.lasso <- penalized(form,data=octrain.dummy,model="cox",
            lambda1=4,lambda2=0) # no L2 penalty
# Ridge regression
fit.ridge <- penalized(form,data=octrain.dummy,model="cox",
            lambda1=0,lambda2=3) # no L1 penalty
```

TABLE 8.1
Oral cancer study. Shown are the hazard ratios of an unpenalized and three penalized Cox regression models. Compared to the first column, all hazard ratios are systematically closer to one (no effect). These are results from complete case analysis (n=456) where all patients with a missing value in at least one variable were removed.

Variable	unpenalized	ridge	LASSO	elastic net
age	1.04	1.04	1.04	1.04
tumorthickness	0.97	0.98	1.00	1.00
genderMale	0.98	0.98	1.00	1.00
tobaccoNever	1.06	1.06	1.00	1.03
deep.invasionYes	1.96	1.85	1.67	1.77
siteFloor.of.Mouth	1.05	1.00	1.00	1.00
siteHard.Palate	5.51	1.53	1.00	1.01
siteLower.Gum	0.48	0.50	0.56	0.53
siteRetromolar.Trigone	1.08	1.02	1.00	1.00
siteTongue	1.19	1.09	1.00	1.05
siteUpper.Gum	3.24	1.55	1.00	1.09
raceNonCauc	0.86	0.93	1.00	0.99
x.posnodes	1.14	1.14	1.14	1.14
tumormaxdimension	1.17	1.17	1.15	1.16
vascular.invasionYes	1.68	1.58	1.45	1.52

Each of the four Cox regression models whose hazard ratios are shown in Table 8.1 can be used to predict the individualized risks of death within 5 years. Table 8.2 shows specific predictor variable values that characterize a hypothetical patient. Table 8.3 shows the predicted 5-year risks of death when the hypothetical patient is diagnosed with cancer at different ages.

TABLE 8.2
Oral cancer study. Shown are the predictor variable values that characterize a
hypothetical patient for whom we compute the predicted 5-year risks in Table
8.3 and Panel B Figure 8.4.

Predictor variable	Predictor value
tumorthickness	0.9
genderMale	1.0
tobaccoNever	1.0
deep.invasionYes	0.0
siteFloor.of.Mouth	1.0
siteHard.Palate	0.0
siteLower.Gum	0.0
siteUpper.Gum	0.0
siteRetromolar.Trigone	0.0
siteTongue	0.0
x.posnodes	2.0
raceNonCauc	0.0
tumormaxdimension	2.0
vascular.invasionYes	1.0

TABLE 8.3
Oral cancer study. The predicted 5-year risk of death (%) of the unpenalized
Cox regression and the three penalized Cox regression models whose hazard
ratios are shown in Table 8.1. The first column shows the age in years, the
other variables were fixed at the values shown in Table 8.2. The second column
shows the predicted risk of the benchmark null model (Kaplan-Meier method)
which does not depend on age (or any other predictor variable).

Age	Null model	Unpenalized	ridge	LASSO	Elastic net
29.0	46.7	23.1	22.7	22.6	22.7
40.0	46.7	32.6	31.8	31.4	31.6
63.0	46.7	60.5	58.3	56.9	57.7
74.0	46.7	75.3	72.7	71.0	72.0
80.0	46.7	82.5	80.0	78.3	79.3

This illustrates how much the predicted risks of the three penalized Cox regression models deviate from the predicted risk of the unpenalized Cox regression in selected patient profiles. Due to the shrinkage of the hazard ratios toward zero, it seems natural that the predicted risks are shrunk toward the predicted risk of the null model (Kaplan-Meier method) which does not include any predictor variables. To verify this intuition, it is useful to illustrate how the regression coefficients (in this case hazard ratios), and correspondingly, the individualized predicted risk, change according to increasing values of the penalty parameters. Panel A of Figure 8.4 shows the so-called regularization paths for the LASSO model of Table 8.1. With increasing penalty, the hazard ratios are all shrunk toward the value 1 (no effect). Panel B of Figure 8.4 shows that the subject-specific predicted risk of the penalized model converges to the predicted risk of the null model (Kaplan-Meier method) which ignores the predictor variables.

Next, we need to discuss the task of choosing the values of the penalty parameter. In order to build the best prediction model, the choice of the penalty parameter needs to be integrated into the modeling algorithm [20]. One level of cross-validation is needed to choose the value of the penalty parameter. To illustrate this step of the model-building algorithm, Figure 8.5 shows the prediction performance of different values of the penalty parameter obtained by repeating 5-fold cross-validation 5 times in the learning dataset. Shown are the area under the curve (AUC) and the Brier score for the 5-year prediction time horizon for different values of the LASSO penalty. We see a clear maximum for the AUC and a clear minimum for the Brier score. In this example, the optima of the AUC and Brier score are achieved at the same value of the penalty parameter. If the Brier and AUC scores were not in agreement, we would prefer the Brier score as it reflects both discrimination and calibration (Chapter 5).

```
# R-code
# sequence of candidate penalty values
penalities <- c(0.01,10,100,1000)
# sequence of fitted LASSO models
fit.penal <- lapply(penalities,function(pen){
  fit <- penalizedS3(form,data=octrain.dummy,model="cox",
          lambda2=0,lambda1=pen,trace=FALSE)
  fit$call$lambda1 <- eval(pen)
  fit
})
# cross-validated Brier score and AUC
x.steps <- Score(fit.penal, formula=Surv(survtime,survstatus)~1,
        seed=9, # random seed
        data=octrain.dummy, # training data
        times=60, # prediction time horizon
        split.method="cv5",# 5-fold cross-validation
        B=5) # repeated 5 times
```

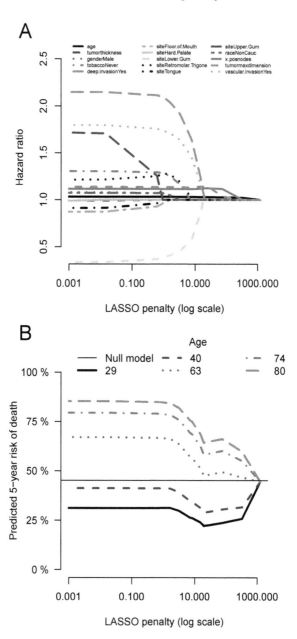

FIGURE 8.4

Panel A shows Park & Hastie [138] regularization paths. Each line represents
the hazard ratio of one of the 15 covariates in the Cox regression model for
increasing LASSO parameter values. On the left border of the x-axis, where
the penalty approaches zero, the hazard ratios approach the hazard ratios of
the unpenalized model. Panel B shows the predicted risks of a sample patient
at different ages characterized by the predictor variable values shown in Table
8.2. The horizontal line is the 5-year risk prediction of the null model.

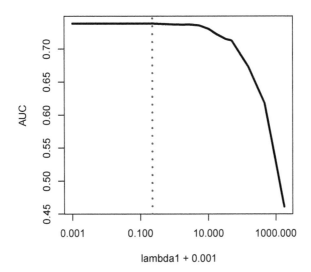

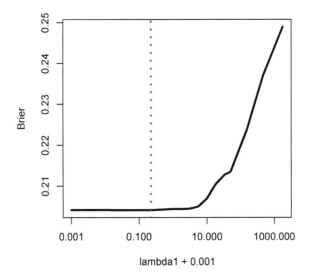

FIGURE 8.5

Choosing the LASSO penalty parameter according to the AUC and Brier score obtained by repeating 5-fold cross-validation 5 times in the learning dataset of the oral cancer study. The dotted vertical lines indicate the value of lambda1 that achieves the optimal performance (maximum AUC and minimum Brier score).

8.2.2   Supervised spline selection

Restricted cubic splines were discussed in Section 4.3.2 as a tool to allow for a non-linear relationship between a continuous predictor variable and the linear predictor of a logistic or Cox regression model. When using this method one needs to choose the number of knots and place them somehow on the scale of the continuous predictor variable: the more knots, the more flexible the relationship.

In Section 8.1, we have argued that expert opinion should guide the selection of the number of knots. Instead, we can let the data decide and *tune* the number of knots. Here it is useful to simultaneously shrink the regression coefficients corresponding to the spline in order to avoid overfitting (Figure 8.6). To let the computer automatically select the number of knots and a corresponding optimal penalty parameter, we could integrate a grid search into the modeling algorithm as follows. We vary the number of knots for each continuous predictor, say from 0 to 5. At the same time we also vary the penalty parameter across multiple candidate values. For each combination of the numbers of knots and the penalty parameter, we calculate the cross-validated Brier score and choose the combination and corresponding penalized regression model with the best prediction performance.

8.3   Machine learning (two levels of cross-validation)

Sometimes we cannot (or do not want to) define the prediction model solely by using subject matter knowledge and a pre-specified formula which dictates how the variables affect the predicted risk. With machine learning we let the data find the formula and extensively use the computer to identify the best model.

A typical machine learning approach uses bootstrap or cross-validation to tune an algorithm that learns from the data. Each machine learning technique has its own set of tuning parameters as we will detail below for some selected methods. To choose the tuning parameters we need a second level of cross-validation for the model building. (Hence, a third, outer layer of cross-validation is needed to evaluate the prediction performance.) There are many different machine learning algorithms [185, 12], but not all come with their fully developed extension for right-censored time-to-event outcome.

It is easiest to think about the advantages and disadvantages of machine learning methods by first envisioning a prediction space (Figure 8.7, Panel A).

In this type of figure, we have two continuous predictor variables along the X and Y axes, and the space in the plot shows the distribution of predicted risks. A logistic regression model, without interactions and without restricted cubic splines, can only assign graded risks along the two axes (Figure 8.7, Panel

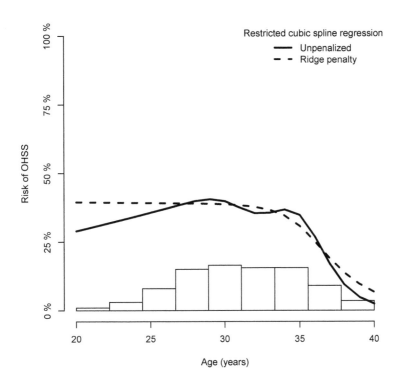

FIGURE 8.6
In vitro fertilization study. Predicted risk of ovarian hyperstimulation syndrome (OHSS) based on two logistic regression models. The unpenalized model is the same as shown in Figure 4.7. The penalized model adds a ridge penalty. Both models estimate a restricted cubic spline to describe a non-linear effect of patient age. The histogram shows the marginal distribution of age in the training set.

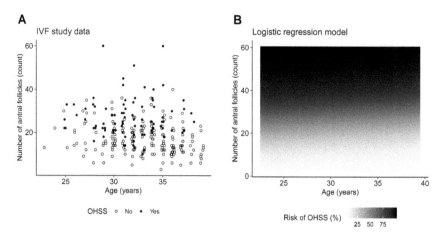

FIGURE 8.7
In vitro fertilization study. Panel A shows the ovarian hyperstimulation syndrome (OHSS) outcome according to age and antral follicle count. Panel B shows the predicted risk of a logistic regression model which assumes linear additive effects of age and antral follicle count on the risk of OHSS.

B). Tree-based methods have the advantage that they can draw numerous lines, but each must be perpendicular to either the X or Y axis (Figure 8.8). Artificial neural networks are even more flexible, in that they can potentially (depending upon how they are constructed) draw a large number of lines or curves (Figure 8.12). So, clearly, classification trees and neural networks are more flexible than logistic regression. However, this flexibility is what gets the methods into trouble. Too much partitioning of the predictor space is a bad thing and will produce suboptimal prediction for future observations [110]. Therefore, machine learning methods all have protocols that attempt to keep them from overfitting or underfitting. Yet, it may require an experienced user and extensive tuning before this works well in practice. The bottom line is that systematic reviews have suggested that machine learning methods predict less accurately than traditional statistical methods [107].

Clearly a (completely pre-specified) logistic or Cox regression model is easier to explain and illustrate than a black box artificial neural network.

Data-dependent variable and functional form selection turns standard regression models into black boxes too.

Moreover, a logistic or Cox regression model has the advantage that it will always give you the same answer when applied to the same dataset. Some machine learning methods use random seeds in the fitting and tuning process and as such can produce different models with different results even when

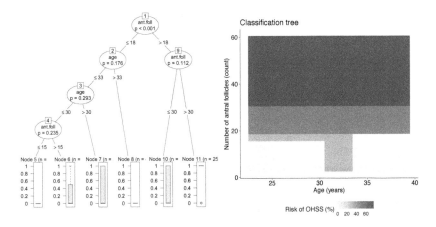

FIGURE 8.8

In vitro fertilization study. The classification tree (left panel) assigns different predicted risks only to 4 different regions (right panel). The regions are defined by thresholds of age and antral follicle count.

applied to the same dataset. Machine learning methods are furthermore prone to produce biologically implausible models as we demonstrate below.

8.3.1   Random forest

A *random forest* [31] is a recommendable machine learning technique which can be used to build risk prediction models with binary, right-censored survival [102], and competing risk outcomes [104]. A forest consists of trees; apart from that there are several versions/implementations of the random forest methodology [125, 101, 84, 184] and each comes with a set of tuning parameters [28, 155].

In our context, the simplest possible tree is a medical test which, based on a predictor variable and a cut-off value, classifies patients as low risk or high risk. An example is the definition of hypertension, which classifies patients as high risk when their systolic blood pressure value is above 140 mmHg. The choice of the threshold is supervised in the sense that the outcome data are used to implement the best possible combination of predictor variable and corresponding threshold in order to optimize the prediction performance.

Admittedly, the simplicity of a single classification tree to demonstrate a prediction model is very appealing (Figure 8.8, Panel A). However, the resulting prediction model (Figure 8.8, Panel B) is biologically implausible: Why would the risk in the case of low antral follicle count increase from 0.0% to 28.5% exactly when patient age changes from 30 to 31 and decrease back to zero exactly when the patient's age changes from 33 to 34?

Another problem with classification trees is that they are highly sensitive to small perturbations of the data. By perturbation of data we mean, for example, removing 10% of the data. Figure 8.9 shows prediction models obtained by recursive partitioning (classification tree) of three bootstrap datasets. The bootstrap datasets contain many different replications of a subject, and in particular, they differ with respect to which subjects are not included (out-of-bag).

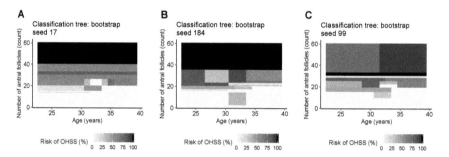

FIGURE 8.9
In vitro fertilization study. The three panels show the predicted risks of classification trees obtained in three bootstrap datasets sampled with replacement from the full data. The random seed used to draw the bootstrap sets is shown in the titles.

It is clear that single patients, for example a patient with age 32 and 22 antral follicles, would receive considerably different predicted risks according to the three tree models shown in panel A, B and C of Figure 8.9. More generally, a prediction model algorithm is called a *weak learner* if it is unstable in the sense that a small perturbation of the data may change the predicted risks considerably. *Bagging* is the idea of creating a *strong learner* by averaging many *weak learners* obtained in bootstrap samples [29]. A random forest is an algorithm which averages many classification trees (an ensemble of trees) obtained in bootstrap samples to construct a *strong learner*. Figure 8.10 shows the individualized risk predictions of two random forest models obtained as follows:

```
# R-code
library(randomForest) # Liaw & Wiener
fit.rf <- randomForest(OHSS~age+ant.foll,data=ivftrain,n.tree=1000)
library(randomForestSRC) # Ishwaran & Kogalur
fit.rfsrc <- rfsrc(OHSS~age+ant.foll,data=ivftrain,n.tree=1000)
```

The good news is that both models are very similar even though they are fitted with different random forest algorithms. The bad news is that they are both biologically implausible: there are small regions with rather low predicted risk inside larger regions with rather high predicted risk and vice versa.

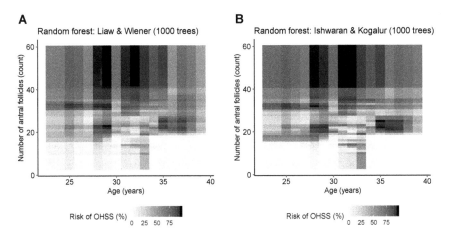

FIGURE 8.10
In vitro fertilization study. Two predictor variables are used to predict the
risk of ovarian hyperstimulation syndrome: age and antral follicle count. The
panels A and B show the predicted risks of two random forest models obtained
with two different implementations of random forest each using 1000 trees and
the default values of all other hyperparameters.

The performance of a random forest can be improved by tuning the number of trees, the number of variables tried at each split and various other
less obvious details of the algorithm. However, the default values of the software often provide reasonable results already [84]. Our illustrative example
depicted in Figures 8.10 is an exception. Here the default values produce risk
prediction models that suffer from overfitting. In addition to being biologically
implausible, as already pointed out above, we see that the models are so badly
calibrated that they have lower predictive performance than the null model
in the test set of the in vitro fertilization study:

```
# R-code
set.seed(98)
fit1 <- rfsrc(OHSS~age+ant.foll,data=ivftrain,n.tree=1000)
set.seed(98)
fit2 <- randomForest(OHSS~age+ant.foll,data=ivftrain,ntree=1000)
x <- Score(list("Ishwaran & Kogalur"=fit1,"Liaw & Wiener"=fit2),
        data=ivftest,formula=OHSS~1,summary="ipa")
summary(x,what="score")
```

Model	AUC (%)	Brier (%)	IPA
Null model	50.0	21.2 [17.6;24.7]	0.0
Ishwaran & Kogalur	68.6 [58.4;78.8]	25.0 [19.0;30.9]	-18.0
Liaw & Wiener	70.1 [60.0;80.2]	22.6 [17.2;27.9]	-6.7

Both models have a negative IPA, meaning that the null model, which ignores the two predictor variables, outperforms the two random forest models. But, why does this happen? It seems that the main reason is that one of the tuning parameters, which is common to all random forest algorithms, is not fully active when there are only two predictor variables. This tuning parameter is the number of predictor variables that is tried each time a mother node is split into two daughter nodes when growing the trees in the bootstrap samples. For a binary outcome, the default value for this hyperparameter is the square root of the total number of predictor variables in both implementations of random forest. So when there are 18 predictor variables, and `mtry` is set to its default value, the `randomForest` algorithm randomly chooses 4 of the 18 variables to identify the next split of the mother node into daughter nodes in the process of fitting the trees to the bootstrap samples. The `rfsrc` algorithm always rounds up and sets `mtry` to 5 by default when there are 18 predictor variables. In our example, the `mtry` parameter is set to 1 by `randomForest` and to 2 by `rfsrc`. So, there is some randomness in the selection of predictor variables for the `randomForest` algorithm but not as much as when there are many predictor variables. But, the randomness in the selection of predictor variables protects the forest against overfitting. This is reflected in the fact that the `randomForest` algorithm scores a less negative IPA value compared to the `rfsrc` algorithm which has no randomness. To investigate this issue further we consider a third random forest algorithm, the `ranger`:

```
# R-code
set.seed(98)
fit3 <- ranger(OHSS~age+ant.foll,data=ivftrain,num.tree=1000,
        probability=1)
x <- Score(list("Wright & Ziegeler"=fit3),
      data=ivftest,formula=OHSS~1,summary="ipa")
summary(x,what="score")
```

Model	AUC (%)	Brier (%)	IPA
Null model	50.0	21.2 [17.6;24.7]	0.0
Wright & Ziegeler	72.7 [63.0;82.4]	19.8 [15.6;24.0]	6.4

We see that with default hyperparameters the `ranger` does not overfit as much as the other two algorithms, because the IPA is positive indicating that the ranger outperforms the null model. A systematic comparison of the default values of the three algorithms quickly shows one important difference: `ranger` sets the minimal node size to 10 whereas `randomForest` and `rfsrc` both set the minimal node size to 1. The minimal node size is the number of unique patients in a terminal node. It is one of several stopping criteria for the tree-building algorithm of a random forest.

To avoid overfitting, the modeler needs to tune the machine learning algorithm.

It is time consuming to provide an overview of tuning parameters for a specific machine learning algorithm, such as random forest. Probst et al. (2019) [149] benchmark random forests based on `ranger`, but they do not consider the other two implementations discussed above. In the present situation, tuning initially means improving the random forest models based on the `randomForest` and `rfsrc` implementations such that they outperform the null model. However, there are many tuning parameters, including but not limited to, the following: the split rule [103], the number of variables tried at each split, the minimal terminal nodesize, the number of trees, the way the bootstrap samples are obtained, the number of variables tried, and the way the terminal nodes are aggregated into a predicted risk.

The idea to tune the minimal node size is motivated by the superior performance of `ranger` compared to `randomForest` and `rfsrc` and the fact that their default minimal nodesize values are different. Thus, we modify the value of the minimal nodesize to see what happens. At minimal nodesize 28, we see that the picture changes dramatically:

```
# R-code
set.seed(98)
fit1 <- rfsrc(OHSS~age+ant.foll,data=ivftrain,n.tree=1000,nodesize
    =28)
set.seed(98)
fit2 <- randomForest(OHSS~age+ant.foll,data=ivftrain,n.tree=1000,
    nodesize=28)
set.seed(98)
fit3 <- ranger(OHSS~age+ant.foll,data=ivftrain,
        num.tree=1000,min.node.size =28,probability=1)
x <- Score(list("Ishwaran & Kogalur"=fit1,"Liaw & Wiener"=fit2,"
    Wright & Ziegeler"=fit3),
        data=ivftest,formula=OHSS~1,summary="ipa")
summary(x,what="score")
```

Model	AUC (%)	Brier (%)	IPA
Null model	50.0	21.2 [17.6;24.7]	0.0
Ishwaran & Kogalur	83.3 [75.3;91.4]	15.8 [12.7;18.8]	25.5
Liaw & Wiener	75.6 [66.4;84.9]	18.2 [13.9;22.5]	14.0
Wright & Ziegeler	76.8 [67.7;85.9]	17.5 [14.1;20.9]	17.4

Next, we tune the nodesize of the three random forest algorithms for our illustrative example given the data that we have. In this situation, tuning of a single hyperparameter means running the algorithm across a search grid of candidate values for this hyperparameter, keeping all other tuning parameters fixed, and using some form of cross-validation of the training data (Section 7.4.3) to choose the value which optimizes the cross-validation performance.

Figure 8.11 shows Brier scores on a grid of candidate nodesizes obtained by repeating 10-fold cross-validation 10 times. Considering this graph, we learn that the three algorithms are apparently optimized at different values for the minimal nodesize, that `rfsrc` does not grow trees when the minimal nodesize exceeds 56, that the optimal value for `ranger` is difficult to find because many values seem to achieve a similar performance, and that `randomForest` has two local optima: one around 10 and another around 80. The latter readily illustrates another nasty hurdle of any tuning task: any attempt to decrease the computational burden, e.g., by intelligently jumping on the search grid of values instead of running through all grid points, is at risk of finding a local optimum instead of the global optimum.

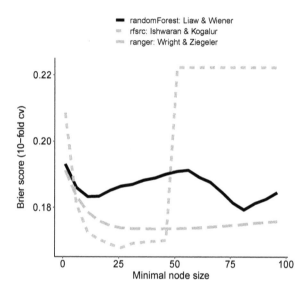

FIGURE 8.11

Tuning of the minimal node size in three different implementations of random forest (`randomForest` by Liaw & Wiener, `rfsrc` by Ishwaran & Kogalur, `ranger` by Wright & Ziegeler). Shown are results of 10 repetitions of 10-fold cross-validation of the learning dataset using 500 trees per forest and all other hyperparameters fixed at their default value.

8.3.2   Deep learning and artificial neural networks

Deep learning is a machine learning approach which was very popular in the context of survival prediction in medical statistics under the alternative name *neural networks* some decades ago [63, 153] and has become popular again [72, 22]. In this rapidly evolving research area, it may be difficult to get an overview of the different algorithms of neural networks and their specific tuning parameters. However, quite generally, the neural network algorithms use the predictor variables to construct new variables called neurons in a number of hidden layers. The first hidden layer defines neurons as linear combinations of the original predictor variables. The neurons of subsequent hidden layers are linear combinations of the neurons of the previous layer. Non-linearity is introduced into the algorithm by means of activation functions, such as the logistic function. Also, the outcome is linked to the last hidden layer by a suitable activation function. The number of hidden layers and the number of neurons per hidden layer are specific to the application at hand. At this point, it is important to emphasize that, when the aim is to build a risk prediction model with artificial neural networks, one should try to introduce prediction performance metrics wherever possible in order to tune the algorithm to guide the construction of layers and to balance the number of hidden layers with weight decay (penalty-driven regularization similar to ridge regression). It is beyond our scope and perhaps not even possible in great generality to define a fully equipped neural networks algorithm that automatically selects a useful medical risk prediction model based on a dataset. Instead, we want to make a different highly important point: a neural network algorithm may lead to a biologically implausible risk prediction model. For illustration, we fit a neural network to the training set of our in vitro fertilization study using only age and antral follicle count as input predictor variables. We choose a single hidden layer that consists of five new variables. We are not tuning the model in any way and emphasize that the purpose of this illustration is to explain what potentially is a problem in many applications of artificial neural networks in medical research.

```
# R-code
set.seed(1) # the model depends on the random seed
nn <- neuralnet(ohss ~ age + ant.foll,
        data=ivftrain,
        hidden=5, # tuning parameter
        act.fct = "logistic") # outcome activation function
```

The left panel of Figure 8.12 illustrates the model with its input layer (age, antral follicle count), a hidden layer with 5 neurons, and an outcome layer (ovarian hyperstimulation syndrome). The right panel of Figure 8.12 shows the predicted risk of ovarian hyperstimulation syndrome that individual patients would receive from this model. From a biological perspective, it makes sense to assume that increasing antral follicle count increases the risk of OHSS. However, for any given age, the change of risk shown in the right panel of Figure 8.12 is dropping to almost zero in between moderate/high-risk areas (indicated by the narrow white stripe). It seems that this reflects overfitting. The problem is not simply that an artificial neural network is prone to overfitting, but rather that this overfitting can be difficult to detect, i.e., when the predictor variable space is high dimensional and not 2-dimensional as in our example. Also, it may very well happen that an overfitting artificial neural network (or other machine learning method) scores the best prediction performance on average (IPA, AUC) with a model that is biologically implausible.

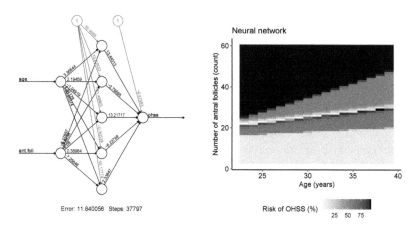

FIGURE 8.12
In vitro fertilization study. The neural network with 1 hidden layer and 5 hidden layer neurons (left panel) assigns different predicted risks to different regions (right panel). The regions are obtained by the resilient backpropagation algorithm with weight backtracking [70].

8.4   The super learner

Even within a single standard regression framework, such as a Cox regression model, there are many alternatives for handling interactions, non-linear effects, and variable selection. Further, one may need to tune hyperparameters such as selecting the amount of shrinkage penalty. With all of these options, it is challenging to know which will be the best in terms of prediction accuracy for future patients. Querying subject matter experts may not fully specify the model, or may lead to a model that asks too much of the data. Naively asking the data for the best model may lead to overfitting. This conundrum is further amplified when one considers that there are other modeling frameworks, such as a random forest. Chapter 6 and Section 7.4 provide tools to select the best model in a list of models. Here we pursue the alternative idea to combine the predictions obtained with a list of risk prediction models into a new, more accurate, risk prediction model.

The super learner uses cross-validation data to combine multiple prediction models into a "super model." From that perspective, the super learner is just another machine learning algorithm which takes in the data and spits out a predicted risk. The super learner is the result of stacking [183, 30, 121] and specifically designed to overcome misspecified regression models and to control all data-dependent modeling steps with cross-validation [176].

Despite the model misspecification concern, another motivation for combining rival modeling algorithms into a new modeling algorithm is as follows. It can happen that the rival models have almost identical prediction performance on average, i.e., in terms of the AUC, Brier score and IPA, but still predict very different risks for individual patients. This is, for example, the case in our oral cancer data examples in Chapter 6 where the performance of the conventional model (Cox regression) is very close to that of the experimental model (random survival forest) at the 10-year prediction time horizon (see Table 6.3). However, Figure 8.13 shows that the two models predict very differently for many patients of the test set. When two strong learners (e.g., Cox regression and random survival forest) disagree about a single subject by much, in particular when one model indicates low risk and the other high risk relative to the overall risk (i.e., the null model prediction), then it seems problematic that one of the two rival models would be used in clinical practice without notice of the discrepancy.

A key element of stacking [183] is the generation of *level-one* data as follows. Leave out the data of a single patient, train a list of strong learners on the remaining data, apply the resulting risk prediction models to the left-out patient, and save the predicted risks together with the outcome of the patient. This generates one row in the level-one dataset. Repeat this with all patients to obtain the full level-one dataset. In the level-one data we have a copy of the outcome of the original (level-zero) data, but instead of the original predictor variables, we have risk predictions, one for each strong learner. Many variations of how to generate the level-one data are possible [183]. For example, to speed up the procedure, one can leave out more than one patient at a time, and train on 9/10 of the data simultaneously to obtain level-one data for the left out 1/10 of the patients.

```
# R-code
fit1 <- cph(Surv(survtime,survstatus)~rcs(age,3)+tumorthickness+
    gender+tobacco+deep.invasion+site+race+x.posnodes+
    tumormaxdimension+vascular.invasion,
        data=octrain.cc, x=TRUE, y=TRUE, surv=TRUE)
set.seed(1972)
fit2 <- rfsrc(Surv(survtime,survstatus)~ age+tumorthickness+gender+
    tobacco+deep.invasion+site+race+x.posnodes+tumormaxdimension+
    vascular.invasion,data=octrain.cc)
x <- Score(list("Cox"=fit1,"Forest"=fit2),
        data=octest.cc,
        formula=Surv(survtime,survstatus)~1,
        times=120,
```

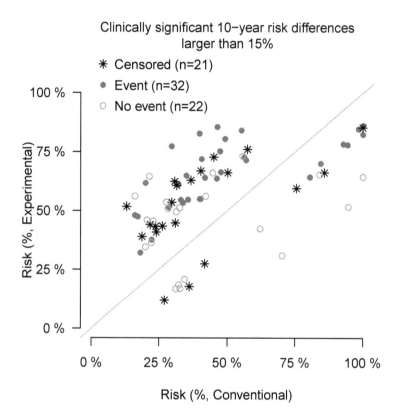

FIGURE 8.13
Oral cancer study. Risk predictions of 10-year mortality for all individuals in the test set where the discrepancy between the conventional and the experimental model is larger than 15%. The risk predicted on the x-axis is a logistic regression model and the risk on the y-axis a random forest model (c.f., Table 6.3).

```
        summary=c("risks"))
level1.data <- dcast(ID ~model,value.var="risk",data=x$risks$score)
level1.data
```

	ID	Null model	Cox	Forest
1:	1	0.6183379	0.4504153	0.5400106
2:	2	0.6183379	0.3953596	0.3126346
3:	3	0.6183379	0.2041489	0.1425181
4:	4	0.6183379	0.5481971	0.3369096
5:	5	0.6183379	1.0000000	0.9843162

264:	264	0.6183379	0.4631094	0.4687943
265:	265	0.6183379	0.1693142	0.1763019
266:	266	0.6183379	0.4381540	0.6954035
267:	267	0.6183379	0.3966399	0.2518442
268:	268	0.6183379	0.5548072	0.4351919

*One can learn from the discrepancies of strong risk prediction models
and implement a new risk prediction model which combines the rivals
in a clever way: the super learner.*

A super learner is obtained by "learning" on the level-one data. One way
to do this is the cross-validation winner-takes-all strategy. The prediction performance is calculated for each column of the level-one data separately and the
best model is chosen. This cross-validation selector has also been called the
discrete super learner [147]. However, Wolpert [183] argues that one should
think about the level one data as any other data. From that perspective the
winner-takes-all strategy corresponds to selecting the best of several risk factors by univariate modeling, whereas combining the risk predictions somehow
corresponds to multiple risk factor modeling. Most often we would prefer the
multiple risk factor model.

Specifically, a super learner is a risk prediction model that exploits the
discrepancies in the risk predictions of a list of rival models and combines
their risk predictions into a weighted average. As with all machine learning
approaches, there are variants of the super learner. The overall idea is to select
a list of modeling algorithms (sometimes called libraries). There are no restric-
tions concerning which modeling algorithms to include in the list other than
software availability. Then, k-fold cross-validation is applied to each modeling
algorithm separately to generate new predictor variables that contain, for each
patient, the predicted risks obtained by applying the algorithms to the fold
where this patient is left out of the modeling. When there are five prediction
modeling algorithms, then five new predictor variables are constructed. It remains to combine the new predictor variables, which contain individualized
risk predictions from the individual models, into a new predicted risk. This is
what Wolpert [183] calls "black art." Breiman proposed to find the best inter-
polating predictor [30] using ridge regression on the level-one data to account

for the correlation of the new predictor variables. Also, the super learner [146] is the weighted interpolation with the highest cross-validation performance.

In this way, the risk prediction of the super learner for a single patient will often be between the most extreme risk predictions obtained with the list of models for this patient. Thus, the super learner solves the problem when equally accurate (same AUC, same Brier score, same IPA) learners (e.g., Cox regression and Random Forest) produce very different probabilities for the same individual patient. In addition, the method has nice theoretical properties [176]. On the downside, we recognize that due to the dependence on cross-validation the super learner result is random which may or may not depend crucially on the random seed.

To illustrate the super learner we use the training data of the in vitro fertilization study and combine a logistic regression model (glm) with a random forest (randomForest) and a neural network (nnet) into a super learner.

```
# R-code
library(SuperLearner)
set.seed(17) # the result depends on the random seed
fit <- SuperLearner(Y=ivftrain[["ohss"]],X=ivftrain[,c("age","ant.
    foll")],SL.library=c("SL.glm","SL.randomForest","SL.nnet"),
    family="binomial")
fit$coef
```

TABLE 8.4
With this particular random seed, the super learner attaches most weight to the logistic regression model (glm) and some weight to the random forest (randomForest) and artificial neural network model (nnet), respectively.

Algorithm	Weight
Model: glm	70.8%
Model: randomForest	19.1%
Model: nnet	10.1%

Table 8.5 shows the test set prediction performance comparing the super learner with the ingredient algorithms. The table is obtained as follows.

```
# R-code
fit1 <- glm(OHSS~age+ant.foll,data=ivftrain,family="binomial")
set.seed(2)
fit2 <- randomForest(OHSS~age+ant.foll,data=ivftrain,ntree=1000,
    importance=0)
set.seed(3)
fit3 <- predict(nnet(OHSS~age+ant.foll,data=ivftrain,size=2),
    newdata=ivftest)
set.seed(4)
SL.fit <- SuperLearner(Y=ivftrain[["ohss"]],
```

```
                X=ivftrain[,c("age","ant.foll")],
                SL.library=c("SL.glm","SL.randomForest","SL.nnet"),
                family="binomial")
fit4 <- predict(SL.fit,newdata=ivftest[,.(age,ant.foll)])$pred
x <- Score(list("Logistic regression"=fit1,"Random Forest"=fit2,"
    Neural net"=fit3,"super learner"=fit4),
        data=ivftest,formula=OHSS~1,summary="ipa")
summary(x,what="score")
```

In this particular scenario, with only two continuous predictors and this particular split of the full data into training and validation sets, the super learner has lower prediction performance than the best model which is the logistic regression model. Nevertheless, the mathematical theory tells us that, in large samples, the super learner is expected to outperform or at least not perform worse than the best of the individual learners [176].

TABLE 8.5
In vitro fertilization study. Test set results comparing the individual risk prediction modeling algorithms with the super learner.

Model	AUC (%)	Brier (%)	IPA
Null model	50.0	21.2 [17.6;24.7]	0.0
Logistic regression	87.8 [81.0;94.7]	13.9 [10.7;17.1]	34.5
Random Forest	70.9 [60.9;80.9]	22.2 [16.9;27.4]	-4.8
Neural net	79.1 [72.0;86.3]	15.2 [12.0;18.3]	28.3
super learner	81.5 [73.4;89.6]	16.6 [12.7;20.6]	21.4

To illustrate what happens when the super learner is applied in practice we consider a single new patient at age 25 with 17 antral follicles. The predicted risks of ovarian hyperstimulation syndrome for this patient are shown in Table 8.6. The predicted risk of the super learner is simply the sum of the predicted risks of the three models weighted according to the values shown in Table 8.4.

```
# R-code
p <- predict(fit,newdata=data.frame(age=25,ant.foll=17))
p
```

In contrast to most other ensemble machine learning methods, including random forest and boosting, which build a prediction model based on many weak learners, the super learner builds a model based on several or many strong learners. In fact, a machine learning model, e.g., obtained with random forest, can be included as one of the strong learners in the super learner library. This means that it requires one layer of cross-validation more than the most layers required for any of the included learners to estimate the prediction performance of the super learner.

TABLE 8.6

Predicted risks of ovarian hyperstimulation syndrome for a 25-year-old patient with 10 antral follicles obtained with logistic regression (`glm`), random forest (`randomForest`), an artificial neural network model (`nnet`) and super learner.

Model	Predicted.risk
Model: glm	26.8
Model: randomForest	32.0
Model: nnet	56.8
super learner	30.8

9

Things you might have expected in our book

9.1 Threshold selection for decision making

Thresholds for decision making shape the busy clinical routine. Humans in charge of decision making like to have clear "if-then-else" instructions. However, when it comes to critical decisions with costs and benefits, a more appropriate and modern way of communicating evidence-based research results is to invoke a risk calculator and to use the result as one important factor for decision making. Smartphone apps are perfectly suited to make this transition happen.

Still, the optimal threshold question is frequently asked, and it is also frequently answered, even though the data sources often do not support it, or the analysis methods are ad hoc [186]. From a purely statistical point of view, we note that estimators of optimal threshold values are notoriously unstable. This is reflected in wide confidence intervals even with large sample sizes. But, how would a confidence interval enter into the decision process? Anyway, taking away 10% of the learning data, or switching from one statistical method to another, should not affect important medical decisions in a black-or-white manner.

Biology is graded and not binary [181]. Medical decisions based on thresholds ignore this fact. Hypertension (too high blood pressure) is just one example. Patients are called hypertensive if they have a systolic blood pressure measurement above 140. However, Kannel et al. [109] looked at this through their Framingham study glasses and concluded that "It is the level of BP that kills, not arbitrarily defined hypertension."

Deriving a threshold which is good for most patients should further depend on costs and benefits of wrongly deciding for or against treatment. More generally, we believe that the level of the predicted risk, where the transition between treatment and no treatment happens, should generally be the result of a doctor-patient interaction, accounting for the predicted risk as one important factor guiding the decision.

The ROC curve, its competitors [97], and also decision curve analysis [182] are tools that commonly consider all possible thresholds simultaneously. Many methods to find the "optimal" thresholds have been proposed, and most of them combine sensitivity, specificity, outcome prevalence and utility in a clever way. An example is Youden's index, which is simply the sum of sensitivity and specificity and the value 1. However, using one of these tools to oversimplify the situation departs from evidenced-based research and is unlikely to be optimal for an individual patient.

9.2   Number of events per variable

A frequently asked question regarding prediction model development is, "how large of a dataset do I need?" A popular response to this question is to examine the events per variable and then apply a rule of thumb. Originally, this was based on some epidemiology research that was related but not exactly prediction model-specific [41], and the rule of thumb became to multiply the number of variables in the model by 10 to obtain the required number of events. So, if you had 8 predictor variables, you would need a cohort (for time-to-event outcome) that contained at least 80 events. The rule was modified to events per model degree of freedom, recognizing that more parameters are estimated when binary variables become those with more than 2 levels or continuous with particular enhancements (e.g., restricted cubic splines) [88]. While this rule of thumb is very easy to apply, recent work [152] has shown that it is not terribly reliable as a rule. Sometimes, having fewer than 10 events per model degree of freedom is okay (i.e., the prediction model still works fine). Other times, more than 10 events per model degree of freedom are actually required. In other words, the situation is more complex than simply the ratio of events to model complexity. For this reason, we are not advocating the events per variable or model degree of freedom concept in this book. Instead, we have discussed penalized regression techniques in Section 8.2.1 which allow us to include all predictor variables.

9.3   Confidence intervals for predicted probabilities

Many clinicians and statisticians adamantly demand that confidence intervals are placed around predicted probabilities to indicate the uncertainty in the prediction. While this is an understandable position to take, in practice, the use of confidence intervals is not all that helpful [112].

The main reason for the limited usefulness of confidence intervals for predicted probabilities lies with interpretation. They are not specific to an individual patient. Rather, they apply to a hypothetical scenario involving the situation where the experiment and estimation process are repeated an infinite number of times. This discrepancy between an individual patient and the correct interpretation of a confidence interval causes the statements typically used to be either vague or incorrect. For example, a patient might be told that his true risk lies within a 95% confidence interval. What does that even mean? Why use the 95% confidence interval, rather than some other choice, say the 91% interval? Alternatively, a patient might be told that his risk is between the lower and upper limits of the 95% confidence interval. The same concerns apply here. In short, there is no sentence that makes sense to the individual patient and correctly interprets the 95% confidence interval.

9.4   Models developed from case-control data

Although elegant methodology has been derived for estimating the absolute risk stemming from case-control studies [19, 119], this type of analysis, when the aim is to make a risk prediction model, is tricky and beyond the scope of our book. We refer to the recent monograph by Pfeiffer & Gail [144] for further reading.

9.5   Hosmer-Lemeshow test

It is not uncommon to see a Hosmer-Lemeshow test reported to assess the calibration of a risk prediction model [100]. In its most common form, the test compares observed event proportions to the average predicted risk within each risk decile. The type-1 error is when the prediction model is calibrated but the test rejects. The type-2 error is where the test claims that the model is calibrated when it is not. In this situation, what is more important: type-1 or type-2 error?

We do not find this test particularly useful. The test has been developed to test goodness of fit, and therefore, it is typically applied to the training data without cross-validation. Another problem is that the test requires that the predictions be grouped with no guidance of how many groups to select, and deciles (a common choice) may be inappropriate in small and in large datasets. However, the result of the test will usually be very sensitive to how the groups are chosen. In small samples, this test is very unlikely to detect miscalibration. In large samples, even slight miscalibration can trigger a significant test of miscalibration. No attention is paid to the clinical significance of the miscalibration.

9.6   Backward elimination and stepwise selection

We strongly discourage analysts from using backward elimination, forward selection, and any other form of stepwise variable selection, see Section 2.7.10 for the reasons. As an alternative, one should use a more sophisticated algorithm, such as penalized regression controlled by cross-validation (Section 8.2.1).

9.7   Rank correlation (c-index) for survival outcome

An extremely popular measure for the performance of a prediction model applied to survival data is a rank correlation coefficient called the c-index (or concordance index) [88]. For a pair of patients where one dies earlier than the other, the c-index is the probability that the one who died first had received the higher predicted risk of dying. Thus, this metric is suitable for evaluating the predictions of event time. However, predictions of event time are seldom of interest, and as such, not covered in our book.

More importantly, the c-index has several drawbacks when used to evaluate the performance of statistical models that predict the probability of an event occurring within a given time horizon. First, the c-index is not what is called a proper scoring rule (see Section 2.2.1) for predicting the t-year risks [26]. Theoretically, the scoring rule used should identify the actual data-generating model as the best model. To see this, consider the following example. We are scoring the data-generating model and a rival model produced by multiplying the data-generating model predictions by a random number. If the scoring rule were to identify the rival model as better than the data-generating model, the scoring rule is not "proper." This is somewhat of a theoretical issue since, in practice, we are never really working with the data-generating model but it remains an important property for a scoring rule to possess.

A second concern with the c-index in this setting is that the horizon time does not enter into the calculation of the score. For example, assume we have a test set with three variables: the predicted probability of an event within 5 years, time to the event, and event status. The fact that the horizon is 5 years does not affect the calculation of the c-index, whereas it should to reflect the situation properly. A third concern, which is basically a restatement of the second concern, is that the event status at the horizon does not, per se, affect the c-index calculated value. All this makes the c-index insensitive to the horizon of interest, such that a Cox proportional hazard model will have the same c-index for 2-year and 5-year predicted risks.

9.8 Integrated Brier score

With time-to-event outcome, the integrated Brier score is obtained by cumulating the Brier score (Chapter 5) across a sequence of prediction time horizons. Usually the prediction time horizons are data driven, i.e., the event times of the subjects in the purpose dataset, and are, as such, not related to a concrete prediction model framework (Section 2.1). The integrated Brier score can be a useful summary of performance when the purpose of the analysis is to compare modeling algorithms with a single number, and the target of the actual prediction is the whole absolute risk curve (whole survival curve in settings without competing risks).

9.9 Net reclassification index and the integrated discrimination improvement

The *integrated discrimination improvement* (IDI) and the *net reclassification index* (NRI) have been proposed to measure the incremental prognostic value that a new marker will have when added to an existing statistical prediction model [140]. Both measures are not recommended to be used because they lack an important property: they are not proper measures of prediction performance [98, 141]. In particular, poorly calibrated models may appear to be "better" than well-calibrated models when performance is measured with either IDI or NRI. One might then proceed to say that one can only use these measures when the models are well calibrated [122]. However, the following easy-to-replicate simulation study demonstrates the severity of the problem with NRI. To illustrate, consider the in vitro fertilization study and a logistic regression model which uses age and antral follicle count. We then computer-simulate 200 independent random noise variables, i.e., 200 "new markers," such that they are useless because they are independent of the outcome (OHSS: ovarian hyperstimulation syndrome) and the two predictor variables. We measure the gain of predictive performance with the NRI, IDI, Δ AUC, and Δ Brier score. Note that we fit the logistic regression models with and without the "new markers" to a small training sample which includes data from only 50 patients. We do this because, in small samples, adding a variable which is not related to the outcome to a logistic regression model leads to minor but systematic over-estimation of the effect sizes of the other predictor variables. Next, we evaluate the performance in the test set. Both the NRI and IDI seem to pick up the over-estimation and associate an increase of predictive performance with way too many of the 200 noise markers, whereas both Δ AUC and Δ Brier associate a decrease of predictive performance with the majority of the noise markers (Figure 9.2).

```
# R-code
B <- 200
ivftrain.small <- ivftrain[sample(1:NROW(ivftrain),size=50)]
result <- foreach(s=1:B,.combine="rbind")%dopar%{
  set.seed(s)
  # function rnorm generates normal noise
  ivftrain.small[,newMarker:=rnorm(NROW(ivftrain.small))]
  ivftest[,newMarker:=rnorm(NROW(ivftest))]
  fit1 <- glm(ohss~ant.foll+age,data=ivftrain.small,family="
    binomial")
  fit2 <- glm(ohss~ant.foll+age+newMarker,data=ivftrain.small,
    family="binomial")
  x <- Score(list("Conventional model"=fit1,"Random marker"=fit2),
          data=ivftest,
          se.fit=0,
          formula=ohss~1)
  library(Hmisc) # provides IDI and NRI
  p1 <- predictRisk(fit1,newdata=ivftest)
  p2 <- predictRisk(fit2,newdata=ivftest)
  y <- improveProb(p1,p2,ivftest$ohss)
  data.table(NRI=100*y$nri,
          IDI=100*y$idi,
          delta.AUC=100*x$AUC$contrasts$delta.AUC,
          delta.Brier=-100*x$Brier$contrasts$delta.Brier[3])
}
boxplot(result,names=c("NRI",
                "IDI",
                expression(paste(Delta,"AUC")),
                expression(paste(Delta,"Brier"))))
abline(h=0,col=2)
```

A more systematic simulation study has shown that even the model that actually generates the data (and as such is the best possible model) can be "improved" by random noise when NRI is used to measure improvement [141].

Much of the attraction of IDI and NRI, by basic scientists, is that these metrics amplify the presumed improvement coming from a new marker, quite possibly making the marker appear to add substantial value when it does not.

9.10   Re-classification tables

Re-classification tables summarize the findings of NRI. To begin, the analyst defines clinically meaningful risk strata. They show counts of re-classified pa-

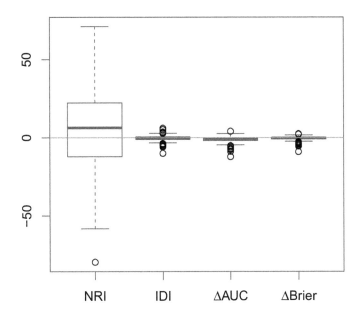

FIGURE 9.1
In vitro fertilization study. Effects of adding a random noise variable to a logistic regression model measured by improper measures, IDI and NRI, and by proper measures, Δ AUC and Δ Brier score. The boxplots show results of repeatedly adding a random noise variable to a logistic regression model (200 times).

tients when changing from one risk prediction model to another, for example, changing from the full model to the model without a marker of interest. While the overall re-classification table is immediately useful, the obvious temptation is to consider the table conditional on the outcome, but this has the same problem as the NRI: a less calibrated model can appear superior to a better calibrated model. To illustrate this problem we again use the in vitro fertilization study where we fit a logistic regression model to the training data with age and antral follicle count as predictors. This is our conventional model. Our exaggerated model is obtained by manipulating the conventional model without adding any additional information as follows. We compute the overall disease prevalence in the training dataset. Our exaggerated model simply assigns 100% predicted risk for all patients whose conventional risk prediction is above the overall prevalence and 0% for the patients where the conventional risk prediction is below the overall prevalence. We then apply both the conventional model and the exaggerated model to the test set patients.

```
# R-code
library(PredictABEL) # provides the re-classification table
OHSSprevalence <- mean(ivftrain$OHSS=="Yes")
# conventional model
fit1 <- glm(OHSS~ant.foll+age,data=ivftrain,family="binomial")
# exaggerated model
fit2 <- function(risk,prevalence){
  new.risk <- risk
  # set risk to 100% when risk is above prevalence
  new.risk[risk>prevalence] <- 1
  # set risk to 0% when risk is below prevalence
  new.risk[risk<=prevalence] <- 0
  new.risk
}
# apply models to test set
p1 <- predictRisk(fit1,newdata=ivftest)
p2 <- fit2(p1,OHSSprevalence)
reclassification(data=ivftest,
        cOutcome=10,
        p1,
        p2,
        cutoff=c(0,.25,.5,.75,1))
```

```
----------------------------------------

   Reclassification table

----------------------------------------

Outcome: absent

                 Updated Model
Initial Model [0,0.25) [0.25,0.5) [0.5,0.75) [0.75,1]  % reclassified
```

[0,0.25)	43	0	0	0	0
[0.25,0.5)	12	0	0	12	100
[0.5,0.75)	0	0	0	3	100
[0.75,1]	0	0	0	1	0

Outcome: present

		Updated Model			
Initial Model	[0,0.25)	[0.25,0.5)	[0.5,0.75)	[0.75,1]	% reclassified
[0,0.25)	3	0	0	0	0
[0.25,0.5)	2	0	0	11	100
[0.5,0.75)	0	0	0	11	100
[0.75,1]	0	0	0	4	0

Combined Data

		Updated Model			
Initial Model	[0,0.25)	[0.25,0.5)	[0.5,0.75)	[0.75,1]	% reclassified
[0,0.25)	46	0	0	0	0
[0.25,0.5)	14	0	0	23	100
[0.5,0.75)	0	0	0	14	100
[0.75,1]	0	0	0	5	0

NRI(Categorical) [95% CI]: 0.6029 [0.3483 - 0.8575] ; p-value: 0
NRI(Continuous) [95% CI]: 1.2267 [0.9029 - 1.5505] ; p-value: 0
IDI [95% CI]: 0.3342 [0.2067 - 0.4616] ; p-value: 0

We see that the tables suggest that the exaggerated model reclassifies many of the test set patients correctly, and IDI and both versions of NRI are significant. However, this cannot be correct because we have not added information.

When NRI or IDI are used to measure prediction performance, then the predictive performance of a conventional model can be "increased" without adding information.

Both the Δ AUC and Δ Brier score indicate that the exaggerated model is worse than the conventional model in the test set patients.

```
# R-code
x <- Score(list("Conventional model"=p1,"Exaggerated model"=p2),
        data=ivftest,
        se.fit=0,
        null.model=FALSE,
        formula=ohss~1)
summary(x)
```

```
$score
              Model AUC (%) Brier (%)
1: Conventional model    87.8     13.9
2:  Exaggerated model    80.7     20.6


$contrasts
              Model          Reference delta AUC (%) delta Brier (%)
1: Exaggerated model Conventional model      -7.1558             6.7
```

Of course this is an extremely exaggerated model to illustrate the point, but slight exaggeration happens easily when adding markers to existing models, and the miscalibration will not be as easy to detect as with our example. Anyway, we conclude that only the combined re-classification table can be interpreted without extreme care.

9.11   Boxplots of rival models conditional on the outcome

In Chapter 5, we use boxplots to illustrate the distribution of a model's predicted risks conditional on the outcome. It is tempting to also use boxplots to visualize differences between rival models conditional on the outcome at the prediction time horizon. However, unfortunately, such boxplots suffer the same problems as their discretized counterpart, the re-classification tables (Section 9.10). We modify the exaggerated model slightly to illustrate the problem. Instead of exaggerating to 100% and 0% we only increase and decrease the conventional risk prediction by 25% according to the overall disease prevalence. The boxplots imply a benefit of the exaggerated model as both the risk of the event-free patients is decreased and the risk of the cases with OHSS is increased. However, since we have not introduced any new information to create our exaggerated model, this model cannot be better, and the boxplots are not to be trusted.

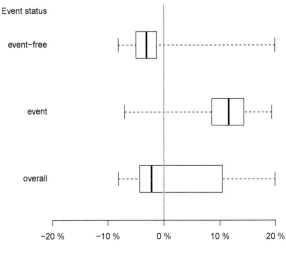

FIGURE 9.2
In vitro fertilization study. Effects of manipulating a conventional logistic
regression model to predict more extreme values. No information has been
added to the conventional, only the predicted risks above the training set
prevalence were increased by 25% and the predicted risks below were decreased
by 25%.

Bibliography

[1] OO Aalen and S Johansen. An empirical transition matrix for non-homogeneous Markov chains based on censored observations. *Scandinavian Journal of Statistics*, 5:141–150, 1978.

[2] Werner Adler and Berthold Lausen. Bootstrap estimated true and false positive rates and ROC curve. *Computational Statistics & Data Analysis*, 53(3):718–729, 2009.

[3] Safina Ali, Frank L Palmer, Changhong Yu, Monica DiLorenzo, Jatin P Shah, Michael W Kattan, Snehal G Patel, and Ian Ganly. A predictive nomogram for recurrence of carcinoma of the major salivary glands. *JAMA Otolaryngology–Head and Neck Surgery*, 139(7):698–705, 2013.

[4] Analytics Vidhya Content Team. Practical guide to deal with imbalanced classification problems in R. https://www.analyticsvidhya.com/blog/2016/03/practical-guide-deal-imbalanced-classification-problems/, Mar 2016.

[5] Per Kragh Andersen, Ørnulf Borgan, Richard D Gill, and Niels Keiding. *Statistical Models Based on Counting Processes*. New York: Springer, 1993.

[6] Per Kragh Andersen, Ronald B Geskus, Theo de Witte, and Hein Putter. Competing risks in epidemiology: Possibilities and pitfalls. *International Journal of Epidemiology*, 41(3):861–870, 2012.

[7] Per Kragh Andersen and Niels Keiding. Multi-state models for event history analysis. *Statistical Methods in Medical Research*, 11(2):91–115, 2002.

[8] Per Kragh Andersen and Niels Keiding. Interpretability and importance of functionals in competing risks and multistate models. *Statistics in Medicine*, 31(11-12):1074–1088, 2012.

[9] Per Kragh Andersen and Maja Pohar Perme. Pseudo-observations in survival analysis. *Statistical Methods in Medical Research*, 19(1):71–99, 2010.

[10] Donna P Ankerst, Josef Hoefler, Sebastian Bock, Phyllis J Goodman, Andrew Vickers, Javier Hernandez, Lori J Sokoll, Martin G Sanda,

John T Wei, Robin J Leach, et al. Prostate cancer prevention trial risk calculator 2.0 for the prediction of low-vs high-grade prostate cancer. *Urology*, 83(6):1362–1368, 2014.

[11] Donna P Ankerst, Johanna Straubinger, Katharina Selig, Lourdes Guerrios, Amanda De Hoedt, Javier Hernandez, Michael A Liss, Robin J Leach, Stephen J Freedland, Michael W Kattan, et al. A contemporary prostate biopsy risk calculator based on multiple heterogeneous cohorts. *European Urology*, 74(2):197–203, 2018.

[12] Susan Athey and Guido Imbens. Machine learning methods economists should know about. *arXiv preprint arXiv:1903.10075*, 2019.

[13] Peter C Austin and Ewout W Steyerberg. The integrated calibration index (ici) and related metrics for quantifying the calibration of logistic regression models. *Statistics in Medicine*, 38(21):4051–4065, 2019.

[14] Peter C Austin and Jack V Tu. Automated variable selection methods for logistic regression produced unstable models for predicting acute myocardial infarction mortality. *J Clin Epidemiol*, 57(11):1138–46, 2004.

[15] Jonathan Bartlett and Ruth Keogh. *smcfcs: Multiple Imputation of Covariates by Substantive Model Compatible Fully Conditional Specification*, 2018. R package version 1.3.1.

[16] Jonathan W Bartlett, Shaun R Seaman, Ian R White, and James R Carpenter. Multiple imputation of covariates by fully conditional specification: Accommodating the substantive model. *Statistical Methods in Medical Research*, 24(4):462–487, 2015.

[17] Jacques Benichou and Mitchell H Gail. Estimates of absolute cause-specific risk in cohort studies. *Biometrics*, pages 813–826, 1990.

[18] Jacques Benichou and Mitchell H Gail. Methods of inference for estimates of absolute risk derived from population-based case-control studies. *Biometrics*, 51(1):182–194, 1995.

[19] Jacques Benichou and Mitchell H Gail. Methods of inference for estimates of absolute risk derived from population-based case-control studies. *Biometrics*, pages 182–194, 1995.

[20] Axel Benner, Manuela Zucknick, Thomas Hielscher, Carina Ittrich, and Ulrich Mansmann. High-dimensional Cox models: The choice of penalty as part of the model building process. *Biometrical Journal*, 52(1):50–69, 2010.

[21] Kasper Drimer Berg, Ben Vainer, Frederik Birkebaek Thomsen, M Andreas Roeder, Thomas Alexander Gerds, Birgitte Groenkaer Toft, Klaus

Brasso, and Peter Iversen. Erg protein expression in diagnostic specimens is associated with increased risk of progression during active surveillance for prostate cancer. *European Urology*, 66(5):851–860, 2014.

[22] Elia Biganzoli, Patrizia Boracchi, and Ettore Marubini. A general framework for neural network models on censored survival data. *Neural Networks*, 15(2):209–218, 2002.

[23] Harald Binder and Martin Schumacher. Adapting prediction error estimates for biased complexity selection in high-dimensional bootstrap samples. *Statistical Applications in Genetics and Molecular Biology*, 7(1), 2008.

[24] P. Blanche, J-F Dartigues, and H. Jacqmin-Gadda. Estimating and comparing time-dependent areas under receiver operating characteristic curves for censored event times with competing risks. *Statistics in Medicine*, 32(30):5381–5397, 2013.

[25] Paul Blanche, Thomas A Gerds, and Claus T Ekstrøm. The Wally plot approach to assess the calibration of clinical prediction models. *Lifetime Data Analysis*, 25(1):150–167, 2019.

[26] Paul Blanche, Michael W Kattan, and Thomas A Gerds. The C-index is not proper for the evaluation of t-year predicted risks. *Biostatistics*, 2018.

[27] Paul Blanche, Cecile Proust-Lima, Lucie Loubere, Claudine Berr, Jean-Francois Dartigues, and Helene Jacqmin-Gadda. Quantifying and comparing dynamic predictive accuracy of joint models for longitudinal marker and time-to-event in presence of censoring and competing risks. *Biometrics*, 71(1):102–113, 2015.

[28] Anne-Laure Boulesteix, Silke Janitza, Jochen Kruppa, and Inke R König. Overview of random forest methodology and practical guidance with emphasis on computational biology and bioinformatics. *Wiley Interdisciplinary Reviews: Data Mining and Knowledge Discovery*, 2(6):493–507, 2012.

[29] Leo Breiman. Bagging predictors. *Machine Learning*, 24(2):123–140, 1996.

[30] Leo Breiman. Stacked regressions. *Machine Learning*, 24(1):49–64, 1996.

[31] Leo Breiman. Random forests. *Machine Learning*, 45(1):5–32, 2001.

[32] Leo Breiman. Statistical modeling: The two cultures. *Statistical Science*, 16(3):199–215, 2001.

[33] Norman E Breslow. Analysis of survival data under the proportional hazards model. *International Statistical Review/Revue Internationale de Statistique*, pages 45–57, 1975.

[34] Glenn W Brier. Verification of forecasts expressed in terms of probability. *Monthly Weather Review*, 78:1–3, 1950.

[35] Ewen Callaway, David Cyranoski, Smriti Mallapaty, Emma Stoye, and Jeff Tollefson. The coronavirus pandemic in five powerful charts. *Nature*, 579(7800):482–483, 2020.

[36] James Carpenter and Michael Kenward. *Multiple imputation and its application*. John Wiley & Sons, 2012.

[37] Weijie Chen, Frank W Samuelson, Brandon D Gallas, Le Kang, Berkman Sahiner, and Nicholas Petrick. On the assessment of the added value of new predictive biomarkers. *BMC Medical Research Methodology*, 13(1):98, 2013.

[38] SC Cheng, Jason P Fine, and LJ Wei. Prediction of cumulative incidence function under the proportional hazards model. *Biometrics*, pages 219–228, 1998.

[39] SC Cheng, LJ Wei, and Z Ying. Predicting survival probabilities with semiparametric transformation models. *Journal of the American Statistical Association*, 92(437):227–235, 1997.

[40] Karl Claxton. The irrelevance of inference: A decision-making approach to the stochastic evaluation of health care technologies. *Journal of Health Economics*, 18(3):341–364, 1999.

[41] John Concato, Peter Peduzzi, Theodore R Holford, and Alvan R Feinstein. Importance of events per independent variable in proportional hazards analysis I. Background, goals, and general strategy. *Journal of Clinical Epidemiology*, 48(12):1495–1501, 1995.

[42] Nancy R Cook, Nina P Paynter, Charles B Eaton, JoAnn E Manson, Lisa W Martin, Jennifer G Robinson, Jacques E Rossouw, Sylvia Wassertheil-Smoller, and Paul M Ridker. Comparison of the Framingham and Reynolds risk scores for global cardiovascular risk prediction in the multiethnic women's health initiative. *Circulation*, 125(14):1748–1756, 2012.

[43] John B Copas. Regression, prediction and shrinkage. *Journal of the Royal Statistical Society: Series B (Methodological)*, 45(3):311–335, 1983.

[44] John B Copas. Using regression models for prediction: Shrinkage and regression to the mean. *Statistical Methods in Medical Research*, 6(2):167–183, 1997.

[45] Giuliana Cortese and Per K Andersen. Competing risks and time-dependent covariates. *Biometrical Journal*, 52(1):138–158, 2010.

[46] Giuliana Cortese, Thomas A Gerds, and Per K Andersen. Comparing predictions among competing risks models with time-dependent covariates. *Statistics in Medicine*, 32(18):3089–3101, 2013.

[47] David R Cox. Regression models and life tables. *Journal of the Royal Statistical Society*, B 34:187–220, 1972.

[48] David R Cox. Partial likelihood. *Biometrika*, 62:269–276, 1975.

[49] Urania Dafni. Landmark analysis at the 25-year landmark point. *Circulation: Cardiovascular Quality and Outcomes*, 4(3):363–371, 2011.

[50] Jan De Neve and Thomas A Gerds. On the interpretation of the hazard ratio in Cox regression. *Biometrical Journal*, page doi: 10.1002/bimj.201800255, 2019.

[51] Liesbeth C De Wreede, Marta Fiocco, and Hein Putter. The mstate package for estimation and prediction in non-and semi-parametric multi-state and competing risks models. *Computer Methods and Programs in Biomedicine*, 99(3):261–274, 2010.

[52] Elizabeth R DeLong, David M DeLong, and Daniel L Clarke-Pearson. Comparing the areas under two or more correlated receiver operating characteristic curves: A nonparametric approach. *Biometrics*, 44(3):837–845, 1988.

[53] Olga V Demler, Michael J Pencina, and Ralph B D'Agostino Sr. Misuse of DeLong test to compare AUCs for nested models. *Statistics in Medicine*, 31(23):2577–2587, 2012.

[54] Thomas G Dietterich. Approximate statistical tests for comparing supervised classification learning algorithms. *Neural Computation*, 10(7):1895–1923, 1998.

[55] Kjell A Doksum and Miriam Gasko. On a correspondence between models in binary regression analysis and in survival analysis. *International Statistical Review/Revue Internationale de Statistique*, pages 243–252, 1990.

[56] Kjell A Doksum and Miriam Gasko. On a correspondence between models in binary regression analysis and in survival analysis. *International Statistical Review/Revue Internationale de Statistique*, 58(3):243–252, 1990.

[57] Bradley Efron. Estimating the error rate of a prediction rule: Improvement on cross-validation. *Journal of the American Statistical Association*, 78(382):316–331, 1983.

[58] Bradley Efron. The estimation of prediction error: Covariance penalties and cross-validation. *Journal of the American Statistical Association*, 99(467):619–632, 2004.

[59] Bradley. Efron and Robert. Tibshirani. Improvement on cross-validation: The .632+ bootstrap method. *Journal of the American Statistical Association*, 92:548–560, 1997.

[60] Hillel J Einhorn and Robin M Hogarth. Behavioral decision theory: Processes of judgement and choice. *Annual Review of Psychology*, 32(1):53–88, 1981.

[61] Claus Thorn Ekstrøm, Thomas Alexander Gerds, and Andreas Kryger Jensen. Sequential rank agreement methods for comparison of ranked lists. *Biostatistics*, 20(4):582–598, 2019.

[62] Frank Eriksson, Torben Martinussen, and Søren Feodor Nielsen. Large sample results for frequentist multiple imputation for cox regression with missing covariate data. *Annals of the Institute of Statistical Mathematics*, pages 1–28, 2019.

[63] David Faraggi and Richard Simon. A neural network model for survival data. *Statistics in Medicine*, 14(1):73–82, 1995.

[64] Julian J Faraway. Does data splitting improve prediction? *Statistics and Computing*, 26(1-2):49–60, 2016.

[65] Tom Fawcett. An introduction to ROC analysis. *Pattern Recognition Letters*, 27(8):861–874, 2006.

[66] Jason Fine and Robert J Gray. A proportional hazards model for the subdistribution of a competing risk. *Journal of the American Statistical Association*, 94(446):496–509, 1999.

[67] Peter Flom. Stopping stepwise: Why stepwise selection is bad and what you should use instead. https://towardsdatascience.com/stopping-stepwise-why-stepwise-selection-is-bad-and-what-you-should-use-instead-90818b3f52df, Sep 2018.

[68] Marie-Cécile Fournier, Etienne Dantan, and Paul Blanche. An r2-curve for evaluating the accuracy of dynamic predictions. *Statistics in Medicine*, 37(7):1125–1133, 2018.

[69] Jerome Friedman, Trevor Hastie, and Rob Tibshirani. Regularization paths for generalized linear models via coordinate descent. *Journal of Statistical Software*, 33(1):1, 2010.

[70] Stefan Fritsch, Frauke Guenther, and Marvin N. Wright. *neuralnet: Training of Neural Networks*, 2019. R package version 1.44.2.

[71] Brian F Gage, Carl van Walraven, Lesly Pearce, Robert G Hart, Peter J Koudstaal, BSP Boode, and Palle Petersen. Selecting patients with atrial fibrillation for anticoagulation. *Circulation*, 110(16):2287–2292, 2004.

[72] Michael F Gensheimer and Balasubramanian Narasimhan. A simple discrete-time survival model for neural networks. *arXiv preprint arXiv:1805.00917*, 2018.

[73] TA Gerds, TH Scheike, and PK Andersen. Absolute risk regression for competing risks: interpretation, link functions, and prediction. *Statistics in Medicine*, 31:3921–3930, 2012.

[74] TA Gerds and M Schumacher. Consistent estimation of the expected Brier score in general survival models with right-censored event times. *Biometrical Journal*, 48(6):1029–1040, 2006.

[75] TA Gerds and M Schumacher. On Efron type measures of prediction error for survival analysis. *Biometrics*, 63:1283–1287, 2007.

[76] TA Gerds and MA van de Wiel. Confidence scores for prediction models. *Biometrical Journal*, 53(2):259–274, 2011.

[77] Thomas A Gerds, Per Kragh Andersen, and Michael W Kattan. Calibration plots for risk prediction models in the presence of competing risks. *Statistics in Medicine*, 2014.

[78] Thomas A Gerds, Tianxi Cai, and Martin Schumacher. The performance of risk prediction models. *Biometrical Journal*, 50(4):457–479, 2008.

[79] Thomas Alexander Gerds. The Kaplan-Meier theatre. *Teaching Statistics*, 38(2):45–49, 2016.

[80] Jelle J Goeman. L1 penalized estimation in the Cox proportional hazards model. *Biometrical journal*, 52(1):70–84, 2010.

[81] Ted A Gooley, Wendy Leisenring, John Crowley, and Barry E Storer. Estimation of failure probabilities in the presence of competing risks: New representations of old estimators. *Statistics in Medicine*, 18(6):695–706, 1999.

[82] Erika Graf, Claudia Schmoor, and Martin Schumacher. Assessment and comparison of prognostic classification schemes for survival data. *Statistics in Medicine*, 18:2529–2545, 1999.

[83] Sander Greenland, James M Robins, and Judea Pearl. Confounding and collapsibility in causal inference. *Statistical Science*, pages 29–46, 1999.

[84] Ishwaran H and Kogalur UB. *Random Forests for Survival, Regression, and Classification (RF-SRC)*, 2019. R package version 2.9.1.

[85] David J Hand. Evaluating diagnostic tests: The area under the ROC curve and the balance of errors. *Statistics in Medicine*, 29(14):1502–1510, 2010.

[86] James A Hanley and BJ McNeil. A method of comparing the areas under receiver operating characteristic curves derived from the same cases. *Radiology*, 148:839–843, 1983.

[87] Frank E Harrell. *Regression Modeling Strategies. With Applications to Linear Models, Logistic Regression and Survival Analysis.* Springer Series in Statistics. New York, NY: Springer, 2001.

[88] Frank E Harrell, K L Lee, and D B Mark. Multivariable prognostic models: Issues in developing models, evaluating assumptions and adequacy, and measuring and reducing errors. *Statistics in Medicine*, 15:361–87, 1996.

[89] Trevor Hastie, Robert Tibshirani, and Jerome Friedman. *The Elements of Statistical Learning: Data Mining, Inference, and Prediction.* Springer Science & Business Media, 2009.

[90] Walter W Hauck, Sharon Anderson, and Sue M Marcus. Should we adjust for covariates in nonlinear regression analyses of randomized trials? *Controlled Clinical Trials*, 19(3):249–256, 1998.

[91] Walter W Hauck, John M Neuhaus, John D Kalbfleisch, and Sharon Anderson. A consequence of omitted covariates when estimating odds ratios. *Journal of Clinical Epidemiology*, 44(1):77–81, 1991.

[92] Patrick J Heagerty, Thomas Lumley, and Margaret S Pepe. Time-dependent ROC curves for censored survival data and a diagnostic marker. *Biometrics*, 56(2):337–344, 2000.

[93] Ottar Hellevik. Linear versus logistic regression when the dependent variable is a dichotomy. *Quality & Quantity*, 43(1):59–74, 2009.

[94] Michael Henke, Dominik Mattern, Margaret Pepe, Christina Bézay, Christian Weissenberger, Martin Werner, and Frank Pajonk. Do erythropoietin receptors on cancer cells explain unexpected clinical findings? *Journal of Clinical Oncology*, 24(29):4708–4713, 2006.

[95] Miguel A Hernan. Counterpoint: Epidemiology to guide decision-making: Moving away from practice-free research. *American journal of epidemiology*, 182(10):834–839, 2015.

[96] Miguel A Hernan and James M Robins. *Causal Inference.* CRC Boca Raton, FL, 2010.

[97] Jørgen Hilden. The area under the ROC curve and its competitors. *Medical Decision Making*, 11(2):95–101, 1991.

[98] Jørgen Hilden and Thomas A Gerds. A note on the evaluation of novel biomarkers: Do not rely on integrated discrimination improvement and net reclassification index. *Statistics in Medicine*, 33(19):3405–3414, 2014.

[99] Arthur E Hoerl and Robert W Kennard. Ridge regression: Biased estimation for nonorthogonal problems. *Technometrics*, 12(1):55–67, 1970.

[100] David W Hosmer Jr, Stanley Lemeshow, and Rodney X Sturdivant. *Applied Logistic Regression*, volume 398. John Wiley & Sons, 2013.

[101] Torsten Hothorn, Peter Buehlmann, Sandrine Dudoit, Annette Molinaro, and Mark Van Der Laan. Survival ensembles. *Biostatistics*, 7(3):355–373, 2006.

[102] H Ishwaran, UB Kogalur, EH Blackstone, and MS Lauer. Random survival forests. *Annals of Applied Statistics*, 2:841–860, 2008.

[103] Hemant Ishwaran. The effect of splitting on random forests. *Machine Learning*, 99(1):75–118, 2015.

[104] Hemant Ishwaran, Thomas A Gerds, Udaya B Kogalur, RD Moore, SJ Gange, and BM Lau. Random survival forests for competing risks. *Biostatistics*, 15(4):757–773, 2014.

[105] Kristel JM Janssen, Yvonne Vergouwe, A Rogier T Donders, Frank E Harrell, Qingxia Chen, Diederick E Grobbee, and Karel GM Moons. Dealing with missing predictor values when applying clinical prediction models. *Clinical Chemistry*, 55(5):994–1001, 2009.

[106] Nicholas P Jewell. Correspondences between regression models for complex binary outcomes and those for structured multivariate survival analyses. In *Advances in Statistical Modeling and Inference: Essays in Honor of Kjell A Doksum*, pages 45–64. World Scientific, 2007.

[107] MA Jie, Gary S Collins, Ewout W Steyerberg, Jan Y Verbakel, Ben van Calster, et al. A systematic review shows no performance benefit of machine learning over logistic regression for clinical prediction models. *Journal of Clinical Epidemiology*, 2019.

[108] Amy C Justice, Kenneth E Covinsky, and Jesse A Berlin. Assessing the generalizability of prognostic information. *Annals of Internal Medicine*, 130(6):515–524, 1999.

[109] William B Kannel, Ramachandran S Vasan, and Daniel Levy. Is the relation of systolic blood pressure to risk of cardiovascular disease continuous and graded, or are there critical values? *Hypertension*, 42(4):453–456, 2003.

[110] M Kattan. Statistical prediction models, artificial neural networks, and the sophism "I am a patient, not a statistic". *Journal of Clinical Oncology*, 20:885–887, 2002.

[111] Michael W Kattan. Evaluating a new marker's predictive contribution. *Clinical Cancer Research*, 10(3):822–4, 2004.

[112] Michael W Kattan. Doc, what are my chances? A conversation about prognostic uncertainty. *European Urology*, 2(59):224, 2011.

[113] Michael W Kattan, Paul Blanche, and Thomas A Gerds. Boxplots for displaying biomarker values and predicted probabilities for survival outcomes. Submitted to Statistics in Medicine, 2019.

[114] Michael W Kattan, James A Eastham, Alan MF Stapleton, Thomas M Wheeler, and Peter T Scardino. A preoperative nomogram for disease recurrence following radical prostatectomy for prostate cancer. *Journal of the National Cancer Institute*, 90(10):766–771, 1998.

[115] Michael W Kattan and Thomas A Gerds. The index of prediction accuracy: An intuitive measure useful for evaluating risk prediction models. *Diagnostic and Prognostic Research*, 2(1):7, 2018.

[116] MW Kattan. Judging new markers by their ability to improve predictive accuracy. *Journal of the National Cancer Institute*, 95(9):634, 2003.

[117] Edward L Korn, Barry I Graubard, and Douglas Midthune. Time-to-event analysis of longitudinal follow-up of a survey: Choice of the timescale. *American journal of epidemiology*, 145(1):72–80, 1997.

[118] Edward L Korn and Richard Simon. Measures of explained variation for survival data. *Statistics in Medicine*, 9(5):487–503, 1990.

[119] Bryan Langholz and Ørnulf Borgan. Estimation of absolute risk from nested case-control data. *Biometrics*, pages 767–774, 1997.

[120] Saskia Le Cessie and Johannes C Van Houwelingen. Ridge estimators in logistic regression. *Journal of the Royal Statistical Society: Series C (Applied Statistics)*, 41(1):191–201, 1992.

[121] Michael LeBlanc and Robert Tibshirani. Combining estimates in regression and classification. *Journal of the American Statistical Association*, 91(436):1641–1650, 1996.

[122] Maarten JG Leening, Ewout W Steyerberg, Ben Van Calster, Ralph B D'Agostino Sr, and Michael J Pencina. Net reclassification improvement and integrated discrimination improvement require calibrated models: Relevance from a marker and model perspective. *Statistics in Medicine*, 33(19):3415–3418, 2014.

[123] S Lemeshow and D Hosmer. A review of goodness-of-fit statistics for use in the development of logistic regression models. *American Journal of Epidemiology*, 115:92–106, 1982.

[124] Catherine R Lesko and Bryan Lau. Bias due to confounders for the exposure-competing risk relationship. *Epidemiology*, 28(1):20, 2017.

[125] Andy Liaw and Matthew Wiener. Classification and regression by randomforest. *R News*, 2(3):18–22, 2002.

[126] Thomas Lumley, Richard Kronmal, and Shuangge Ma. Relative risk regression in medical research: Models, contrasts, estimators, and algorithms. Technical report, University of Washington, Biostatistics Working Paper Series, 2006.

[127] Ian C Marschner and Alexandra C Gillett. Relative risk regression: Reliable and flexible methods for log-binomial models. *Biostatistics*, 13(1):179–192, 2011.

[128] Guillermo Marshall, Bradley Warner, Samantha MaWhinney, and Karl Hammermeister. Prospective prediction in the presence of missing data. *Statistics in Medicine*, 21(4):561–570, 2002.

[129] Torben Martinussen and Thomas H Scheike. *Dynamic Regression Models for Survival Data*. Springer Science & Business Media, 2007.

[130] Jessina C McGregor, Peter W Kim, Eli N Perencevich, Douglas D Bradham, Jon P Furuno, Keith S Kaye, Jeffrey C Fink, Patricia Langenberg, Mary-Claire Roghmann, and Anthony D Harris. Utility of the chronic disease score and Charlson comorbidity index as comorbidity measures for use in epidemiologic studies of antibiotic-resistant organisms. *American Journal of Epidemiology*, 161(5):483–493, 2005.

[131] Allison Meisner, Chirag R Parikh, and Kathleen F Kerr. Biomarker combinations for diagnosis and prognosis in multicenter studies: Principles and methods. *Statistical Methods in Medical Research*, 28(4):969–985, 2019.

[132] Ulla B Mogensen, Hemant Ishwaran, and Thomas A Gerds. Evaluating random forests for survival analysis using prediction error curves. *Journal of Statistical Software*, 50(11), 2012.

[133] Karel GM Moons, Rogier ART Donders, Theo Stijnen, and Frank E Harrell Jr. Using the outcome for imputation of missing predictor values was preferred. *Journal of Clinical Epidemiology*, 59(10):1092–1101, 2006.

[134] Carvell Nguyen, Brandon Isariyawongse, Changhong Yu, and Michael Kattan. The reduce metagram: A comprehensive prediction tool for

determining the utility of dutasteride chemoprevention in men at risk for prostate cancer. *Frontiers in Oncology*, 2:138, 2012.

[135] Brice Ozenne, Anne Lyngholm Sørensen, Thomas Scheike, Christian Torp-Pedersen, and Thomas Alexander Gerds. riskregression: Predicting the risk of an event using Cox regression models. *R Journal*, 9(2):440–460, 2017.

[136] Layla Parast, Su-Chun Cheng, and Tianxi Cai. Incorporating short-term outcome information to predict long-term survival with discrete markers. *Biometrical Journal*, 53(2):294–307, 2011.

[137] Layla Parast, Su-Chun Cheng, and Tianxi Cai. Landmark prediction of long-term survival incorporating short-term event time information. *Journal of the American Statistical Association*, 107(500):1492–1501, 2012.

[138] Mee Young Park and Trevor Hastie. L1-regularization path algorithm for generalized linear models. *Journal of the Royal Statistical Society: Series B (Statistical Methodology)*, 69(4):659–677, 2007.

[139] Judea Pearl and Dana Mackenzie. *The Book of Why: The New Science of Cause and Effect*. Basic Books, 2018.

[140] MJ Pencina, RB D'Agostino Sr, RB D'Agostino Jr, and RS Vasan. Evaluating the added predictive ability of a new marker: From area under the ROC curve to reclassification and beyond. *Statistics in Medicine*, 27(2):157–172, 2008.

[141] Margaret S Pepe, Jing Fan, Ziding Feng, Thomas Gerds, and Jorgen Hilden. The net reclassification index (NRI): A misleading measure of prediction improvement even with independent test data sets. *Statistics in Biosciences*, 7(2):282–295, 2015.

[142] Margaret Sullivan Pepe, Holly Janes, Gary Longton, Wendy Leisenring, and Polly Newcomb. Limitations of the odds ratio in gauging the performance of a diagnostic, prognostic, or screening marker. *American Journal of Epidemiology*, 159(9):882–890, 2004.

[143] Neil J Perkins, Stephen R Cole, Ofer Harel, Eric J Tchetgen Tchetgen, BaoLuo Sun, Emily M Mitchell, and Enrique F Schisterman. Principled approaches to missing data in epidemiologic studies. *American Journal of Epidemiology*, 187(3):568–575, 2017.

[144] Ruth M Pfeiffer and Mitchell H Gail. *Absolute Risk: Methods and Applications in Clinical Management and Public Health*. CRC Press, 2017.

[145] MF Piepoli, AW Hoes, S Agewall, C Albus, C Brotons, AL Catapano, et al. European guidelines on cvd prevention in clinical practice: the

sixth joint task force of the european society of cardiology and other societies on cvd prevention in clinical practice (constituted by representatives of 10 societies and by invited experts) developed with the special contribution of the european association for cardiovascular prevention & rehabilitation (eacpr). *Eur. Heart J*, 37(29):2315–2381, 2016.

[146] Eric Polley, Erin LeDell, Chris Kennedy, and Mark van der Laan. *SuperLearner: Super Learner Prediction*, 2019. R package version 2.0-26.

[147] Eric C Polley and Mark J Van Der Laan. Super learner in prediction. Technical Report 266, Division of Biostatistics, University of California, Berkeley, 2010.

[148] David Martin Powers. Evaluation: From precision, recall and f-measure to ROC, informedness, markedness and correlation. *Journal of Machine Learning Technologies*, 2:37–63, 2011.

[149] Philipp Probst, Anne-Laure Boulesteix, and Bernd Bischl. Tunability: Importance of hyperparameters of machine learning algorithms. *Journal of Machine Learning Research*, 20(53):1–32, 2019.

[150] Cecile Proust-Lima, Pierre Joly, Jean-Francois Dartigues, and Helene Jacqmin-Gadda. Joint modelling of multivariate longitudinal outcomes and a time-to-event: A nonlinear latent class approach. *Computational Statistics & Data Analysis*, 53(4):1142–1154, 2009.

[151] M Shafiqur Rahman, Gareth Ambler, Babak Choodari-Oskooei, and Rumana Z Omar. Review and evaluation of performance measures for survival prediction models in external validation settings. *BMC Medical Research Methodology*, 17(1):60, 2017.

[152] Richard D Riley, Kym IE Snell, Joie Ensor, Danielle L Burke, Frank E Harrell Jr, Karel GM Moons, and Gary S Collins. Minimum sample size for developing a multivariable prediction model: Part ii-binary and time-to-event outcomes. *Statistics in Medicine*, 2018.

[153] Brian D Ripley and Ruth M Ripley. Neural networks as statistical methods in survival analysis. *Clinical Applications of Artificial Neural Networks*, pages 237–255, 2001.

[154] Anthony S Robbins, Susan Y Chao, and Vincent P Fonseca. What's the relative risk? A method to directly estimate risk ratios in cohort studies of common outcomes. *Annals of Epidemiology*, 12(7):452–454, 2002.

[155] Helene C Rytgaard and Thomas A Gerds. Random forests for survival analysis. *Wiley StatsRef: Statistics Reference Online*, pages 1–8, 2018.

[156] Jaya M Satagopan, Kenneth Offit, William Foulkes, Mark E Robson, Sholom Wacholder, Christine M Eng, Stephen E Karp, and Colin B

Begg. The lifetime risks of breast cancer in Ashkenazi Jewish carriers of brca1 and brca2 mutations. *Cancer Epidemiology and Prevention Biomarkers*, 10(5):467–473, 2001.

[157] JM Satagopan, L Ben-Porat, M Berwick, M Robson, D Kutler, and AD Auerbach. A note on competing risks in survival data analysis. *British Journal of Cancer*, 91(7):1229–1235, 2004.

[158] Leonard J Savage. Elicitation of personal probabilities and expectations. *Journal of the American Statistical Association*, 66:783–801, 1971.

[159] TH Scheike, MJ Zhang, and TA Gerds. Predicting cumulative incidence probability by direct binomial regression. *Biometrika*, 95(1):205–220, 2008.

[160] Shaun R Seaman and Ian R White. Review of inverse probability weighting for dealing with missing data. *Statistical Methods in Medical Research*, 22(3):278–295, 2013.

[161] Joshua M Sharfstein, Scott J Becker, and Michelle M Mello. Diagnostic testing for the novel coronavirus. *JAMA*, 2020.

[162] Noah Simon, Jerome Friedman, Trevor Hastie, and Rob Tibshirani. Regularization paths for Cox's proportional hazards model via coordinate descent. *Journal of Statistical Software*, 39(5):1, 2011.

[163] RM Simon, J Subramanian, MC Li, and S Menezes. Using cross-validation to evaluate predictive accuracy of survival risk classifiers based on high-dimensional data. *Briefings in Bioinformatics*, 12(3):203–214, 2011.

[164] M Sperrin, A Pate, T "Van Staa", GP Martin, N Peek, and I Buchan. Using marginal structural models to adjust for treatment drop-in when developing clinical prediction models. *Statistics in Medicine*, DOI: 10.1002/sim.7913:1–13, 2018.

[165] Jonathan AC Sterne, Ian R White, John B Carlin, Michael Spratt, Patrick Royston, Michael G Kenward, Angela M Wood, and James R Carpenter. Multiple imputation for missing data in epidemiological and clinical research: Potential and pitfalls. *British Medical Journal*, 338:b2393, 2009.

[166] J. Subramanian and R. Simon. An evaluation of resampling methods for assessment of survival risk prediction in high-dimensional settings. *Statistics in Medicine*, 30(6):642–653, 2011.

[167] BaoLuo Sun, Neil J Perkins, Stephen R Cole, Ofer Harel, Emily M Mitchell, Enrique F Schisterman, and Eric J Tchetgen Tchetgen. Inverse-probability-weighted estimation for monotone and nonmonotone missing data. *American journal of epidemiology*, 187(3):585–591, 2017.

[168] BaoLuo Sun and Eric J Tchetgen Tchetgen. On inverse probability weighting for nonmonotone missing at random data. *Journal of the American Statistical Association*, 113(521):369–379, 2018.

[169] Jeremy MG Taylor, Yongseok Park, Donna P Ankerst, Cecile Proust-Lima, Scott Williams, Larry Kestin, Kyoungwha Bae, Tom Pickles, and Howard Sandler. Real-time individual predictions of prostate cancer recurrence using joint models. *Biometrics*, 69(1):206–213, 2013.

[170] Anne Thiebaut and Jacques Benichou. Choice of time-scale in Cox's model analysis of epidemiologic cohort data: A simulation study. *Statistics in Medicine*, 23(24):3803–3820, 2004.

[171] Robert Tibshirani. Regression shrinkage and selection via the LASSO. *Journal of the Royal Statistical Society: Series B (Methodological)*, 58(1):267–288, 1996.

[172] Tue Tjur. Coefficients of determination in logistic regression models – a new proposal: The coefficient of discrimination. *The American Statistician*, 63(4):366–372, 2009.

[173] Célia Touraine, Catherine Helmer, and Pierre Joly. Predictions in an illness-death model. *Statistical Methods in Medical Research*, 25(4):1452–1470, 2016.

[174] Anastasios Tsiatis. *Semiparametric Theory and Missing Data*. Springer Science & Business Media, 2007.

[175] Sean R Tunis, Joshua Benner, and Mark McClellan. Comparative effectiveness research: Policy context, methods development and research infrastructure. *Statistics in Medicine*, 29(19):1963–1976, 2010.

[176] Mark J Van der Laan, Eric C Polley, and Alan E Hubbard. Super learner. *Statistical Applications in Genetics and Molecular Biology*, 6(1), 2007.

[177] Hans van Houwelingen and Hein Putter. *Dynamic Prediction in Clinical Survival Analysis*. CRC Press, 2011.

[178] Hans C Van Houwelingen. Dynamic prediction by landmarking in event history analysis. *Scandinavian Journal of Statistics*, 34(1):70–85, March 2007.

[179] Hans C van Houwelingen and Hein Putter. Comparison of stopped Cox regression with direct methods such as pseudo-values and binomial regression. *Lifetime Data Analysis*, 21(2):180–196, 2015.

[180] Stijn Vansteelandt, James Carpenter, and Michael G Kenward. Analysis of incomplete data using inverse probability weighting and doubly robust estimators. *Methodology*, 6:37–48, 2010.

[181] Andrew J Vickers, Ethan Basch, and Michael W Kattan. Against diagnosis. *Annals of Internal Medicine*, 149(3):200–203, 2008.

[182] Andrew J Vickers and Elena B Elkin. Decision curve analysis: A novel method for evaluating prediction models. *Medical Decision Making*, 26(6):565–574, 2006.

[183] David H Wolpert. Stacked generalization. *Neural Networks*, 5(2):241–259, 1992.

[184] Marvin N Wright and Andreas Ziegler. ranger: A fast implementation of random forests for high dimensional data in C++ and R. *Journal of Statistical Software*, 77(1):1–17, 2017.

[185] Xindong Wu, Vipin Kumar, J Ross Quinlan, Joydeep Ghosh, Qiang Yang, Hiroshi Motoda, Geoffrey J McLachlan, Angus Ng, Bing Liu, S Yu Philip, et al. Top 10 algorithms in data mining. *Knowledge and Information Systems*, 14(1):1–37, 2008.

[186] Laure Wynants, Maarten van Smeden, David J McLernon, Dirk Timmerman, Ewout W Steyerberg, Ben Van Calster, et al. Three myths about risk thresholds for prediction models. *BMC Medicine*, 17(1):192, 2019.

[187] JF Yates. External correspondence: Decompositions of the mean probability score. *Organizational Behavior and Human Performance*, 30(1):132–156, 1982.

[188] Waleed A Yousef, Robert F Wagner, and Murray H Loew. Estimating the uncertainty in the estimated mean area under the ROC curve of a classifier. *Pattern Recognition Letters*, 26(16):2600–2610, 2005.

[189] Qian M Zhou, Wei Dai, Yingye Zheng, and Tianxi Cai. Robust dynamic risk prediction with longitudinal studies. *Statistical Theory and Related Fields*, 1(2):159–170, 2017.

[190] Hui Zou and Trevor Hastie. Regularization and variable selection via the elastic net. *Journal of the Royal Statistical Society: Series B (Statistical Methodology)*, 67(2):301–320, 2005.

Index

Ingram Content Group UK Ltd.
Milton Keynes UK
UKHW022211270423
420857UK00020B/98

9 780367 673734